The Interpretation of Death

EDITED AND INTRODUCED BY
HENDRIK M. RUITENBEEK, Ph.D.

Jason Aronson, Inc., Publishers

for Harry Diaz,
who is full of life.

de lente maakt deuren
de wind is een open hand
wij moeten nog beginnen te leven
HANS LODEIZEN

Library of Congress Catalog Card Number: 73-81214
ISBN: 0-87668-095-3

Manufactured in the United States of America

ACKNOWLEDGMENTS

The editor and publisher have made every effort to determine and credit the holders of copyright of the selections in this book. Any errors or omissions may be rectified in subsequent printings. For permission to use these selections, the editor and publisher make grateful acknowledgment to the following:

"Death and the Pleasure Principle" *by Kurt Eissler:* Reprinted from PSYCHIATRY AND THE DYING PATIENT by Kurt Eissler by permission of International Universities Press.

"Treatment of a Dying Patient" *by Janice Norton:* Reprinted from THE PSYCHOANALYTIC STUDY OF THE CHILD, Volume 18, by permission of International Universities Press.

"On the 'Longing to Die'" *by Kate Friedlander:* Reprinted from the *International Journal of Psycho-Analysis* by permission.

"On 'Dying Together'" and "An Unusual Case of 'Dying Together'" *by Ernest Jones:* Reprinted from ESSAYS IN APPLIED PSYCHO-ANALYSIS by Ernest Jones by permission of International Universities Press and The Hogarth Press Ltd.

"The Psychology of Dying" *by Daniel Cappon:* Reprinted from *Pastoral Psychology*, February 1961 by permission of the Editor and Dr. Daniel Cappon, M.B., F.R.C.P., D.P.M., Toronto, Canada.

"Notes upon the Fear of Death" *by Mary Chadwick:* Reprinted by permission from the *International Journal of Psycho-Analysis*.

"Psychotherapy for the Dying" *by Hattie R. Rosenthal:* Reprinted by permission of the author. Originally published in *American Journal of Psychotherapy*, July 1957.

"Death—The Giver of Life" *by Jordan M. Scher:* Reprinted by permission of the author.

"Psychotherapy and the Patient with a Limited Life-Span" *by Lawrence LeShan and Eda LeShan:* Reprinted by special permission of The William Alanson White Psychiatric Foundation, Inc. from *Psychiatry: Journal for the Study of Interpersonal Processes*, (1961) 24: 319–323. Copyright © 1961 by The William Alanson White Psychiatric Foundation, Inc. Reprinted by permission of the authors.

"Fear of Death" *by Hanna Segal:* Reprinted by permission from the *International Journal of Psycho-Analysis* and by permission of the author.

"The Problem of Death" *by Herman Feifel:* Reprinted from *Catholic Psychological Record*, Volume 3, Spring 1965 by permission of the Editor and the author.

"Death of a Patient During Psychotherapy" *by William H. Young, Jr.:* Reprinted by special permission of the William Alanson White Psychiatric

I take into my arms the death
Maturity exacts,
And name with my imperfect breath
The mortal paradox.
—DONALD HALL,
"My Son, My Executioner"

Preface

The topic of death remains among us as the last, though rapidly fading, taboo. Certainly up until a decade ago the mere discussion of the implications of death both for the dying and living person was considered, if not in bad taste, certainly an issue which had to be avoided at all cost. In all of the professions concerned with medicine and the mental health field almost all participants felt distinctly uncomfortable with the issue of death and dying.

Medical doctors, psychiatrists, and psychoanalysts would avoid the unpleasantness of having to confront the patient with the possibility of dying or prepare relatives for the death of their patients. The denial of death both with patient and doctor was maintained to the very last moment of the actual death.

The appearance of Elisabeth Kubler-Ross' book *On Death and Dying* in 1969 shocked many into the recognition of the fact that a cruel play was being performed upon patients and relatives in not confronting (and preparing) them for the imminent death. The Kubler-Ross book was the beginning of a frank and vivid discussion about the implications of death in our modern society. The book received wide national attention and stimulated others to re-examine their often archaic attitudes towards death and dying.

The collection presented here is in a sense the outcome of that discussion. While many of the papers appeared long before the Kubler-Ross book, they had been ignored by the mental health profession out of their own uneasiness with the topic. No particular solutions are suggested in these papers but they point to the problem of death in our modern society and the plight of the individual when faced with inevitable death.

HMR

CONTENTS

DEATH

MOURNING

Introductory Essay:
REFLECTIONS ON DEATH AND MOURNING

HENDRIK M. RUITENBEEK

"... simplify me when I'm dead." KEITH DOUGLAS

"In de oorlog
In de oorlog hebben we mijn vader in een antieke
kast begraven. Die hebben we toen moeten ge-
bruiken, omdat er geen kisten meer waren te krij-
gen. Wel zonde natuurlijk van zo'n mooie kast."
PAUL VAN SOLINGEN en TOM WEERHEYM
in *Laat je niet kisten**

Death continues to intrigue man. The shock of death never ceases
to amaze us and each time it occurs we wonder and ask ourselves,
"Why?" Reactions to death are manifold. Some express it in
almost violent grief, others in quiet hysteria, and again others
might even laugh. For our reactions are not prescribed, neither
are they predictable. The mystery that surrounds death confronts
us at an early age. I remember from my own childhood that we
were intrigued and curious when we discovered that the curtains
in the windows of one of the houses on our street were all drawn, a
sign that someone had died during the night. We would ask questions as to the nature of what was going on there behind the closed

---

*Translation from the Dutch is as follows:
"During the war
During the war we have buried my father in an antique chest. We had to use
this chest because there were no coffins left. It was such a pity to see that beauti-
ful chest buried."
Paul van Solingen and Tom Weerheym in *Do Not Let Yourself Be Buried in a
Coffin.*"

1

windows. The subject of death was to a large degree taboo as was that of sex and so we were not always able to find out what was going on. But then we would watch the house and see perhaps a coffin being brought in, people in black would enter the house and our parents would go to pay their respects. Finally the tangible evidence appeared when the day of the funeral arrived and all of us would watch the beautiful flower arrangements which were placed on the casket, and there was the wonder of why there were all those flowers, which so much represented the very essence of life.

The paradox had already struck us at that time. But, of course, as children we did not comprehend the totality and finality of death. It created a certain excitement among us[1] and it was something to be curious about, sometimes even to be envious about. I remember that in grade school the father of one of my classmates had suddenly died and, first of all, my friend did not appear for a few days in school (an unexpected vacation!) . Then, when he did come back, he had something special which the others in our class did not have. Obviously, since the teacher gave him more attention and consideration than the rest of us.

Then, growing up, death confronts us increasingly and we see people we know weep over the passing of a relative. We read the poets who are concerned with the problem of death and we try to explain to ourselves and others what our thoughts are about death. A war (in my instance, the Second World War) will bring death in all its grimness to the fore and slowly we begin to realize that death is something which affects us all. Some of us, in sheer astonishment (and sometimes despair), turn to the questions of life, others become even more preoccupied with the notions and implications of death. Some seek out a religion which might console them in denying death[2] or which might even intensify (to the point of terror) the question of death for them.[3] Others try to ignore death altogether. But no one escapes the ultimate confrontation in his own life.

Reactions to the phenomenon of death have long been the subject of intensive study by psychoanalysts. It was Freud who in his classic paper "Mourning and Melancholia" emphasized the psychoanalytic implications for those who were left behind, and I quote:

Now in what consists the work which mourning performs? I do not think there is anything far-fetched in the following representation of it. The testing of reality, having shown that the loved object no longer exists, requires forthwith that all the libido shall be withdrawn from its attachments to this object. Against this demand a struggle of course arises—it may be universally observed that man never willingly abandons a libido-position, not even when a substitute is already beckoning to him.

This process of detachment has not been made easy by the fact that we exalt the dead and again I quote Freud to illustrate this. He writes in his paper "Thoughts on War and Death":

> We suspend criticism of him, overlook his possible misdoings, issue the command: *De mortuis nil nisi bene,* * and regard it as justifiable to set forth in the funeral-oration and upon the tombstone only that which is most favourable to his memory. Consideration for the dead, who no longer need it, is dearer to us than the truth, and certainly, for most of us, is dearer also than consideration for the living.

So the process of proper detachment from the one who has passed away becomes an increasingly difficult one, but it can certainly be worked through in the psychoanalytic process. After all, the psychoanalyst in this instance deals with the problem of life. The patient has to find new ways and patterns of behavior which will put him right back in the midst of life. New attachments have to be established and, although mourning is meaningful, it never should take the place of the initial attachment. The mourning has to be worked through, whereupon the confrontation with life, although it may not be easy and may often be painful, will take its place.

However, the situation is different when the psychoanalyst is confronted with the patient who knows that he is dying. It is probably one of the most difficult tasks a therapist will have to face in the course of his practice. He will need all his skill and compassion to cope with it. There is still relatively little case material on this particular aspect of the psychotherapy of dying. A most moving essay[4] appeared some years ago and the writer, psychotherapist Florence Joseph, relates her experience with a girl dying of cancer. At one time she wrote in a letter to her patient the following:

> Above all do not be ashamed of being a baby. We all regress into

*Of the dead [say] nothing but good.

childhood when we are in deep discomfort and physical pain. I can remember at the birth of my baby calling out to my mother who had been long since dead, "Mummy, where are you?" You must, dear, agree to have nurses around the clock [she had refused three nurses because of the expense, although her brother, who was paying the bills supposedly in the form of a "loan" to her, was urging her to do so]. When you have bad dreams at night, your own nurse must be near at hand, and you should not be left alone. Money can always be made up afterwards. Do not feel guilty at expressing irritation at your mother. She understands, and it would grieve her if she thought you were burdened with remorse on her account. You must feel free to express yourself in any way you wish. You must suppress nothing that gives you any relief, either physically or mentally. Please, dear, do not refuse sometimes to take the sedation that your doctor ordered and that your nurse wishes to give you when you are in pain. It is nonsense to worry that you are becoming dependent on it. I promise you that you will never become a drug addict; when the pain and discomfort cease, you will feel no need of drugs; and some day, Alice, not too long away, this awful discomfort and pain will be over [I hesitated to write this—was it too clear to her?—no, she would take the meaning from it that was best for her]. And in the meanwhile you have the love of your family and of me. You know, poor baby, that I love you.

In this anthology I have included a particularly helpful and beautiful essay by Janice Norton on the same subject. In the discussion of the treatment of the dying patient, one, of course, should not fail to mention Kurt Eissler's book *The Psychiatrist and the Dying Patient,* in which he cites some valuable case material.[5]

As a matter of fact, I selected as the first essay for the section on Death the article by Kurt Eissler on "Death and the Pleasure Principle," in which he discusses the relationship of ego and death and emphasizes that life and death are different aspects of the same process. I was particularly struck by the following statement, which I wish to bring to the attention of the reader:

> Death almost always comes both too early and too late—too early because the ego has rarely realized all of its potentialities, and too late because individual life has been a detour leading finally to what it had been at the beginning: nothingness.

I have already mentioned the second essay in this book, "Treatment of a Dying Patient," which in a most extraordinary manner describes the interaction between the analyst and the patient, which in this instance (since the patient is dying) brings the use of transference to the fore. As Eissler remarks, "It is conceivable that through the establishment of transference, through an approach which mobilizes the archaic trust in the world and reawakens the primordial feelings of being protected by a mother, the suffering of the dying can be reduced to a minimum even in case of extreme physical pain"

Suicide cannot be ignored in the discussion of death, and Kate Friedlander's essay on the "longing to die" is a classic treatise on the subject, where, like Freud, she links suicide to the function of the libido.

Ernest Jones is represented here with two essays, rather neglected by current psychoanalytic literature, in which he discusses suicide in terms of the wish "to die together." He cites a case of a couple who died together at Niagara Falls and links Heinrich von Kleist's suicide to his traveling mania (i.e., to escape with mother).

Daniel Cappon in "The Psychology of Dying" takes a more traditional religious view of dying and cites some material to illustrate his points. The English psychoanalyst Mary Chadwick is represented here with an essay on the fear of death, while Hattie Rosenthal discusses the fear of death in the process of psychotherapy.

A second essay by Hattie Rosenthal is especially concerned with "a psychotherapy for the dying." It has already become a well-known piece in the literature because of its sensitivity and understanding insight.

My friend Jordan Scher gives in his essay "Death—The Giver of Life" a most unusual description and analysis of his encounter with prisoners in Chicago who were condemned to death.

Untimely death still comes as a shock to those who are left behind. But it is even more of a shock when the untimely death is the death of a young person. Samuel Lehrman in his essay is concerned with some of the pathological reactions to this event, their origin and their meaning.

Lawrence LeShan and Eda LeShan discuss in their paper the implications of psychotherapy for patients with a limited life-span. Here all the patients were suffering from cancer.

The treatment in psychotherapy of older patients always will create questions as to the nature and meaning of death. Hanna Segal, a London psychoanalyst, is represented here with a most insightful essay on the analysis of an old man and his fear of dying. Herman Feifel is well-known for his book *The Meaning of Death* and he contributes an essay on the same topic, discussing the problem of death where it concerns the aging person.

William Young in his essay "Death of a Patient During Psychotherapy" sets forth all the anxieties of patient and therapist in the experience of the oncoming death: "'My experience with death and with grief outside therapy, I am sure, enabled me to better deal with my ambivalent feelings toward her impending death, and the experience helped us both to establish the 'community of spirit' which Eissler has pointed out as so necessary for a successful psychotherapeutic experience in this kind of situation."

The English psychoanalyst and sociologist Elliot Jaques concerns himself in his essay "Death and the Mid-Life Crisis" with those who are reaching middle age and for whom death as a reality becomes evident.

Howard Becker, one of this country's most outstanding sociologists, discusses the sorrow of bereavement and the various forms of sorrow in preliterate and literate cultures. The reaction of a young seventeen-year-old toward the death of the mother is discussed in Robert Creegan's remarkable piece "A Symbolic Action During Bereavement."

Melanie Klein, an eminent English psychoanalyst, relates the phenomenon of mourning to manic-depressive states in her patients. Channing Lipson comes back in his contribution, "Denial and Mourning," to Freud's original theses and he discusses in particular the denial of death by those who are left behind.

Harry Slochower treats of the relationship between Eros and the trauma of death in a learned essay. The last essay, by Karl Stern *et al.*, concerns itself with the grief reactions of the elderly and should be most helpful for those who are treating older people who, much more than our younger patients, are confronted with the subject of death and mourning.

NOTES

1. The excitement of the living (and surviving) about death is well illustrated by Paul van Solingen and Tom Weerheym in their Dutch book on funeral customs, where they relate the example of a woman who used to visit all of the funeral parties she could possily go to, because it gave her such "a feeling of excitement," and the woman interviewed even said that she did not need any sex!
2. Christian Science is one of the current religions which try to deny the phenomenon of death altogether.
3. Some of the conservative and extreme Dutch Calvinist groups literally terrify their followers with the notion of death.
4. Florence Joseph, "Transference and Countertransference in the Case of a Dying Patient," in *The Psychoanalytic Review*, Vol. 49, No. 4 (Winter 1962) .
5. See especially case II, on page 154 of Eissler's book (New York: The International Universities Press, 1955) .

DEATH

I. DEATH AND
THE PLEASURE PRINCIPLE

KURT EISSLER

Death is the only event concerning the whole psychobiological organism which is predictable beyond dispute once birth has taken place. Though this is a truism, it is a far-reaching one. Logicians teach that it is wrong to say the sun will rise tomorrow. If we want to be exact, we have to state—so the logician rightly informs us—that the sun will rise tomorrow if the present cosmic conditions are in force at that time. Such a form is necessary if predictions are to be meaningful. Strangely enough, the prediction of the death of organisms is the only prediction which does not require equivalent qualifications. F. C. S. Schiller has correctly disputed the traditional syllogism which leads to the conclusion that Socrates is mortal. Nevertheless, I believe that the mortality of organisms can be predicted without qualification since life and death are different aspects of one and the same process. In strange contradiction to this knowledge, the ego cannot imagine the state of its own death.

Yet man's eternal life can be the content of a thought and can also be imagined in conformity with man's incapacity to imagine death. One feels inclined to say that it is not necessary for man to imagine his own death because it is the only certain event which will occur beyond any dispute. With due permission for teleological thinking, one may find a deep purpose in this incapacity, since, if man could imagine his own death, this might destroy the ego's paramount function as a barrier against the death instinct's premature attainment of its goal.

In other words, would man not make far more frequent use of the capacity of laying hands upon himself if he could really imagine the state of death? In two famous passages allusion was made to this possibility. When Socrates says in the *Apology:* "If you suppose that there is no consciousness, but a sleep like the sleep of him who is undisturbed even by dreams, death will be an unspeakable gain," he expresses the idea which Hamlet, marveling about man's

11

attachment to life, expresses in the reverse: "To sleep, perchance to dream, ay there's the rub." Both seem to agree that the imagination of a state of unconsciousness and its identification with death would have an extreme attractiveness for man.

Socrates and Hamlet disregarded momentarily the fundamental fact that a state of death cannot be imagined. Apparently the ego is inhibited under ordinary circumstances in striving toward a goal which it can represent only in thought but not in its imagination. I am omitting here temporarily the energic aspect of psychoanalysis and have stressed only a fundamental fact of preconscious and conscious functions, whose value, however, must not be underestimated in their great contribution toward impeding the ego's surrender to death. This stress upon the ego's disinclination to strive for the unimaginable will elicit the argument that the state of sleep cannot be imagined either, although the ego gladly tries to attain it. Sleep, however, occurs before an ego has been formed. Furthermore, as has been shown (Anna Freud, 1950), the child struggles against sleep in a certain phase of ego development, namely when he becomes aware of the world of objects and starts to engage himself actively in it. The ego must learn to integrate the biological function of sleep which is fully formed during the initial phases of its development. Only the certainty that the ego will find the world of objects again makes sleep a pleasurable process. The slightest doubt about the prospect of reawakening actually results in grave sleeping disturbances in the adult (Fenichel, 1942). Finally one must mention the ego's unique relationship to this biological function. It is essentially helpless if we disregard the artificial digestion of soporifics. Whereas the ego can actively support and assist the gratification of all other biological needs by effort, irritation, or stimulation, it can do almost nothing in order to induce sleep other than tempting complete exhaustion, which very often is a cover-up for a self-destructive tendency amounting to a suicidal attempt.

The ego's attitude toward death seems ambiguous. Death almost always comes both too early and too late—too early because the ego has rarely realized all of its potentialities, and too late because individual life has been a detour leading finally to what it had been at the beginning: nothingness. This antinomy inherent in man's feeling about death finds its echo in the symbolism with which man has surrounded death: death is at times the redeemer, at times the revenger, then again the force of injustice which kills the young and lets suffer the old; at times he is visualized as the great democrat who does not heed hierarchical superiority or spare the wealthy, the King, and even the Pope. These mutually contradictory feelings about death, which have been found so profusely since Christianity took hold of the Occident, are not universal. A less differentiated ego probably repudiates the idea of death without hesitation or compromise whenever it concerns the self or an unambivalently loved person but welcomes it, again without hesitation or compromise, whenever it concerns the ego-alien, the foreign, the enemy (Freud, 1915a). This clear-cut distribution of positive and negative attitudes toward death can nowadays perhaps be found occasionally in children but not in adults. Feelings of guilt, the mutual penetration of love and hatred, the barriers against the uninhibited discharge of aggression, the deep injuries man's narcissism has suffered by the discoveries of science (Freud, 1917), and many other factors have left their indelible traces upon man's feeling about death although the ancient and primordial abhorrence of it is still noticeable. Yet notwithstanding this abhorrence, there is the remarkable ease with which the ego risks its own destruction in order to achieve its goals. Ambition, competition, the craving for prestige and for adventure lead man often toward exposure to the gravest dangers.

Puzzled, one may ask what the profit of such daring actions may be, if they are so likely to cause death. The frequent recurrence of one pattern inclines us toward considering it a rule: the fear of castration is so great that the destruction of one's self appears preferable. Man's reaction seems to be, with surprising frequency: rather dead than castrated.

Two components of the castration complex are involved. The possession of the penis promises and guarantees the experience of greatest pleasure and the possession of the penis provides also narcissistic gratification. The social area in which man's motivation derives momentum from the castration complex is vast. Almost all those situations in which competition with contemporaries or defeat by others leads to internal situations unbearable for the ego are genetically derivatives of the castration complex. Clinically one can observe that men who have attained relative freedom from the castration complex in their relationship with women still are under its sway in their relationship with men. Freud's description (1937) of the paramount obstacle in the analysis of males finds confirmation in daily observation. The traumatic situation, as is well known, occurred when it dawned on the boy that there are beings who do not possess penises and when he compared the smallness of his organ with the size of that of adult males, further when he feared or wished that the father would make out of him a girl and use him sexually. Here a deep sexual desire comes in conflict with a narcissistic motive, namely, the pride in masculinity (Freud, 1918).

The narcissistic component of the castration complex transgresses its original scope and becomes one of the principal sources of male narcissism. Its later efflorescences are so intensive that many a psychologist overlooks its origin and wants to derive man's main motivation solely from craving for prestige and self-respect. Indeed, many patients are so intensely attached to prestige values that it requires much patience and astuteness in order to obtain also the biological factor (castration complex in the narrower meaning of the term). It is most impressive and likewise puzzling to observe male patients—the same can be easily found in the biographies of nonneurotics—risking their existence in order to make sure of their superiority over competitors. Delinquent patients will destroy their whole careers on the spur of the moment in order to prove to themselves and—in their fantasy—to their environment that they can defy their fathers and are not afraid of them (Fenichel, 1939).

When the intensity of the complex is above average, the variety of social situations which fall within the scope of the castration complex appears to be infinite. What is said here of male psychology is encountered in women in the relationship to the child. Barrenness or loss of a child results, with most women, in a similar conflict as that observed in men when traumatized by an event which unconsciously means castration.

We encounter here a situation of fundamental importance in a discussion of the psychology of death. Apparently man cannot tolerate life without the prospect of pleasure. Concomitantly one can also observe an approximate readiness to die when maximum pleasure is experienced, pleasure which the ego feels cannot be surpassed.

It is my impression that at the height of true orgasm, when for moments the ego is lost, and during the subsequent short time of complete satiation, when the ego is almost inaccessible to external or internal stimulation, a person is ready to surrender to death without struggle (Ferenczi, 1924). The future is then no longer represented and any action of meaning or importance has become inconceivable. In an early phase of psychoanalytic theory, a similar problem played a significant role in regard to the formation of the theory of sexuality. Freud (1905a) emphasized at that time the well-known situations in the lives of some animals who become easy prey when they are in a state of sexual excitement. (I wonder whether the state of defenselessness induced by sleep incurs the same dangers.) Yet this biological situation seems reestablished internally in man when he reaches that level of gratification implicitly inherent in the orgastic capability (Freud, 1909c; Keiser, 1949; Needles, 1953). This constellation is reflected in language. A particular instance occurs in "The Canonization" by John Donne. In the explication of this poem, Cleanth Brooks (1947) makes this point, noting that "in the sixteenth and seventeenth centuries 'to die' means to experience the consummation of the act of love." I feel inclined to believe that this factor also—besides the many other factors usually mentioned—has its bearing upon the fact that in our society most men do not attain the full orgastic peak; the average ego can only tolerate an intensity which is far below the potential maximum.

Likewise I have observed in a few deliveries I have witnessed a brief period in which the woman has been overwhelmed by a passionate triumph incomparable to anything that could be experienced in other circumstances. Here also I had the feeling that in this moment life had reached a peak from which the rest appeared utterly meaningless and negligible. In that moment, perhaps, a woman is also ready to surrender without regret and pain to deprivation of a future. Puerperal depressions may contain (aside from the well-known involvement of aggression and guilt feeling) a deep biological factor arising from the self-evident truth that a woman has reached the maximum of her creative potential in the moment when she has given birth to a living child.

Be this as it may, the fact—which for many may be a truism—that life becomes intolerable without prospect of pleasure contains no small psychological problem. Understandable as it is that only the prospect of pleasure keeps the basic processes of ego formation going, that the transformation of the pleasure principle into the reality principle requires the promise of pleasure pending though postponed, it is difficult to fathom why a mature ego which has integrated the fundamental necessities of life, which has experienced most of the great pleasures life can provide, still needs the prospect of some pleasure in order to continue its existence. I am not speaking here of the pleasure-unpleasure relation in the melancholic patient. I am referring to the basic fabric of the ego which requires the attainment of pleasure if it is to fulfill its functions.

It is most impressive to watch what this ego can achieve. It can go through the greatest deprivations; its capacity to bear pain is incredible; its versatility and sagacity in bending reality to its own purposes are infinite, and again it will not be deterred by maximum sacrifices in fulfilling this function. But all these almost miraculous achievements are based on the prospect of some future pleasure. When this prospect — illusionary or realistic — crumbles, the whole ego organization crumbles likewise and death becomes the only solution, regardless of what the biological life potential of the person may still be. Here the ego, in my estimation, shows quite openly the last vestige of its origin: it shows that it arose totally and completely from drives. Far as it may go in accepting the reality principle, it cannot overstep this last limitation. Boastingly as some may have claimed that they have succeeded in casting off all sources of profane pleasure, that worldly love has lost its meaning, and that all their efforts are absorbed in meditation and contemplation of God, no one—as far as I know—would claim that he could live without pleasure; for in such moments of supreme elevation beyond the world as we know it and of supreme turning toward a deity, the new state implicitly becomes a source of greater pleasure than the individual had known prior to the attainment of that state. And also, the stoics and cynics of ancient antiquity who made themselves independent of the lure of secular pleasures still derived pleasure from this new state of alleged immunity.

The disorder of melancholia has been used as a clinical proof of the existence of a death instinct (Federn, 1930; Weiss, 1935). I believe that this proof is not succinct since the clinical picture is so much complicated by the turning of sadistic drives against the ego (Brun, 1953). I surmise that the clinical fact of the ego's need for pleasure, if it is to function, and the frequent preference of death over castration may be clinical observations preferable to those yielded by the melancholic patient for a discussion of the subject matter. Jones (1927a) introduced the concept of aphanisis into psychoanalytic terminology. He signified with the term a state in which the ego would suffer "the total, and of course permanent, extinction of the capacity (including opportunity) of sexual enjoyment" beyond castration. Castration, if measured by aphanisis, would mean only a partial loss. I believe that the concept of aphanisis is an important one. Its elaboration may lead to a better comprehension of the representation of death in the various psychic systems. Though death cannot be represented in the unconscious, aphanisis can. The anthropological fact (Rivers, 1911) that some peoples do not draw the line between life and death, but between health on one side, sickness and death on the other—as it is expressed in their vocabulary—may support this view. Aphanisis then would include sickness and death, that is to say, all states in which the gain of pleasure is impossible.

In the following I would like to use the term in a way which is different from Jones's. Aphanisis may include the absence of all potentialities of pleasures (the sexual and nonsexual ones) or the absence of all pleasures except those derived from the penis. I am referring here exclusively to male psychology. In women the constellation is far more complicated and less transparent than in men.

We can describe the following clinical alternatives:

(1) The ego may accept aphanisis in order to preserve the penial pleasure, a state one can observe occasionally in perversions where feelings of guilt force the ego to give up all pleasures except the forbidden perversion leading to orgasm.

(2) The ego may accept castration in order to escape aphanisis. Feelings of guilt enforce genital inactivity for the sake of keeping almost all other avenues of pleasure open.

(3) The ego strives for the preservation of all avenues of pleasure, but risks aphanisis, that is to say death, in order to assure the integrity of the penis and superiority over other men. Defeat means castration in such instances and death is preferred.

This third alternative is of interest here. Whatever the imagery of death may mean in the individual instances, the clinical fact remains that often forces which easily lead to self-destruction become activated with a presumptive threat to the penial integrity. I believe we are dealing here with the same destructive forces which would also unfold their deleterious effect if the ego were supposed to function without actual enjoyment or prospect of pleasure. Whether the total deficit of pleasure or its prospect, respectively, would lead to suicide or a psychosis, or a suicide-like exposure to danger, would not make a difference in the context of this discussion. The main point is the sudden damaging effect upon the ego, a damage which is perpetrated by something instinctual in case pleasure is abolished or threatened with abolishment. I believe the clinical observation compels the assumption that one of the functions of the ego is to make innocuous these injurious forces which can be observed clinically as soon as basic pleasure mechanisms are destroyed or threatened with destruction.

II. TREATMENT OF
A DYING PATIENT*

JANICE NORTON

Case reports of dying patients are rare. In 1915 in "Thoughts for the Times on War and Death" Freud discussed our attitude toward death as being "far from straightforward. To anyone who listened to us we were of course prepared to maintain that death was the necessary outcome of life, that everyone owes nature a death and must expect to pay the debt—in short, that death was natural, undeniable and unavoidable. In reality, however, we were accustomed to behave as if it were otherwise. We showed an unmistakable tendency to put death on one side, to eliminate it from life. We tried to hush it up." Considering the universality of the experience of dying, the relative rarity of case material dealing with dying patients would suggest a continued reluctance to deal with dying. Nearly all authors writing of dying patients remark on this (Aronson, 1959; Brodsky, 1959; Eissler, 1955; Feifel, 1959; L. and E. LeShan, 1951; Sandford, 1957; Saul, 1959; Weisman and Hackett, 1961). At the same time they also make a plea for more thorough study of the psychology of dying and insist that the psychiatrist may have a psychotherapeutic role with the dying. Freud (1915, 1916) and Eissler (1955) deal most adequately with both conscious and unconscious reasons for avoiding the dying, and I do not propose to repeat their discussions here.

What follows is a detailed case summary of the last three and a half months of life of a gallant and articulate woman. The case report owes its existence to the fact that all those on whom we usually rely to spare us the necessity of listening to dying patients, family, clergy, friends, other physicians, had already relinquished their roles and could not be induced to resume them. I was faced

*I would like to express my indebtedness to René Spitz, whose ideas and encouragement were invaluable in this case [author's note].

with the choice of allowing this patient to die a miserable and lonely death, possibly by suicide, or of trying to relieve her suffering in so far as I could.

Case Report

Mrs. B., the thirty-two-year old married mother of two sons, five and three, reluctantly came to see me at the urging of her sister, a social worker from a distant city. Her sister had been visiting and had become alarmed at Mrs B.'s increasing depression·and her hints at suicidal thoughts. While the patient frankly told me both were present, she herself felt no need to see a psychiatrist as both depression and a wish to commit suicide seemed to her to be entirely reasonable under the circumstances. She had substantial pain, cough, hemorrhagic tendencies, anemia, and increasing fatigue from metastatic breast cancer; she was losing weight and strength rapidly, had little appetite, slept poorly, and it was apparent to her that X-ray therapy, hormones, and repeated transfusions were having increasingly little effect in controlling the relentless progression of the disease toward her death. She was using very small doses of morphine, mostly at night, in a partial attempt to control the pain and in order to sleep, but had been told to use narcotics very sparingly because of the possibility of addiction. She felt it quite reasonable to wish to stop her suffering by suicide and also felt her suicide would considerably lessen the burden she was imposing on her parents, her sons, and her husband. She told me all this in a quite matter-of-fact way, underscoring the idea that she felt no need to see a psychiatrist and was only coming in once in order to please her sister. She felt she had the right to die as she pleased, had drugs readily available to her, and that her suicide could be made to look like death due to the disease if she took an overdose of morphine at some time when she was unusually sick. She had not confided this plan to anyone, although her statements about her wish to die without a prolonged terminal phase of pain and increasing incapacitation had alarmed her sister; the rest of the family had taken these to mean that she was sick and in pain but "just talking" at times when she felt most uncomfortable.

The breast cancer had been diagnosed very late in the pregnancy with the younger son and a radical mastectomy was performed immediately; following delivery she had bilateral oophorectomy and irradiation to the breast area. She was initially worried about recurrence or spread of the disease, but as several months passed without symptoms she felt encouraged, and except for occasional feelings of regret about the imposed limitation on the size of her family, she was pleased with her life: her husband was enthusiastically beginning his career; her sons were doing well and gave her much pleasure; and she herself was engrossed with her life. Eight months before she came to see me, she had begun to suffer with chest pain and X ray immediately demonstrated metastases to the ribs, spine, and pelvis. Both her husband and surgeon had frankly discussed this with her at her request, and although for about two months she tried to convince herself that X ray and hormones might either cure her or give her "years" yet to live, the steady accumulation of symptoms was more than she could deny. She became very conscious of the fact that death was imminent in the immediately foreseeable future.

She did not become depressed at this point, but instead turned to religion. Her father had been a minister until his recent retirement, and she had been brought up in a religious home. In college she had gradually become more and more intellectually doubting of her faith and had finally lost interest in religion. With the knowledge of her impending death, however, she attempted to return to religion through a Protestant minister whom she engaged in lengthy philosophic discussions, particularly on the subject of immortality. Unfortunately, he took her intellectual arguments at face value, agreed there was no scientific proof of an afterlife and that her doubts were well founded. He offered her faith as a substitute for logic, but this patient, although deeply religious, remained quite skeptical of standard religious doctrine. For several months, however, she continued to find talking with him comforting. Gradually their conversations became more personal and less religious, although occasionally when she was feeling unusually ill he would read to her from the Bible. She became increasingly involved with him and about two months before she came to see me, she had confided to him that she felt she might be falling in love with him. He responded by telling her that this was unrealistic, that she was sick, and by sharply curtailing their time together. In fact, he very shortly stopped seeing her entirely except in a superficial and perfunctory way. Her depression and suicidal preoccupation began at this time. She also became increasingly anxious and had several acute attacks of anxiety, which she attributed to bouts of increased pain and weakness.

Concurrent with this experience were other mounting difficulties in her relationships with important people. She presented everyone with a picture of a young woman visibly dying an early death who had a great need to come to terms with her feelings about this. As subsequent therapy with me bore out, listening had its problems as the entire situation was tragic. She was an appealing, attractive woman, warm, intelligent, well read, interested in many things, and capable of very intense feeling. One result of this was that all who loved her most and might have been expected to help her with her feelings about dying were intensely and understandably involved in grieving. Talking to others of her feelings about dying was virtually precluded by the intensity of the feelings she provoked in them. Her parents, both chronically ill and in their seventies, lived nearby and periodically cared for the children, but they could not bring themselves to see her because they "hated to cry" in her presence. Her husband, increasingly miserable at her impending death, busied himself with his work. Her doctors, increasingly frustrated at her lack of medical response to their various forms of treatment, became hearty and hollow; and her sister, frightened by the patient's obvious loneliness and despair, lived a great distance away and referred her to me. At the time I first saw her, her relationships with the two boys were about all that remained even relatively intact. She had not yet spent any protracted time in the hospital and was using what strength she had to continue to care for them as she always had, although this was becoming an increasing problem for her.

That this patient had remarkable ego strengths was immediately evident. She had faced surgery, pain, sickness, and the knowledge of her impending early death with impressive insistence on reality, and was doing her utmost to adapt to very adverse circumstances. She had continued her life as usual within the limits of her physical condition, did not resort to the drugs readily available to her, and the only demands she had made on those around her were that they allow her to share her experience with them. It was only when she became aware of their increasing withdrawal from her that she became suicidal. Her attitude toward her parents, her husband, and her doctors was essentially maternal, that she was protecting them from pain by not insisting that they listen and help her with her ever-increasing distress. At the same time she was well aware of her need for help and had done her utmost to find it.

Treatment: Early Phase

All of this became apparent in my initial interviews with the patient and, despite her superficial objections to psychiatric treatment, it was possible to get her to continue to see me on a regular basis by agreeing that she had no serious, long-standing psychiatric problems, that she was facing an extraordinarily painful reality situation with admirable courage, but that it might be of some help to her if we were to talk over her feelings about this. In addition, with the relieved consent of her surgeon, I took over the management of her narcotics and sedation so that very soon she became relatively free of pain and began to sleep at night. I explained this to her as essential both for her comfort and for her ability to care for the children as she wished to. She never did agree very wholeheartedly to the idea of seeing a psychiatrist and even in the last week of her life teased me about what an "unpsychiatric psychiatrist" I had been in that I had never lived up to her stereotype of what a psychiatrist should be, a silent, remote interpreter of dreams and of the oedipal situation. The implication was that she had not really had psychiatric treatment but had found someone with whom she could talk, who fortunately happened to be a physician and was, almost by unhappy accident, a psychiatrist as well. My initial treatment plan was to help her with her depression, prevent her suicide if at all possible, and to see if I could help the family to deal with the situation somewhat more effectively. By this time, however, both her husband and her parents had so decathected their relationship with the patient that it proved impossible for them to help; to them, in many respects she was already dead or had in any event delayed her dying too long. Her sister lived too far away to be of any immediate help although she did come to stay with the patient and care for her during the last three weeks of her life. As a result of this, my treatment goal was very rapidly changed to that of trying to make this patient's death less lonely and frightening. To this end, I saw her daily in my office, the hospital, or at her home, depending on her physical condition, for the last three and a half months of her life. I made it explicit that I would be available to her at any time, and would be for as long as she needed me (Eissler, 1955).

She was the older of two girls. Her sister had had training as a social worker, but was happily married and no longer working. Her parents were hardworking, well meaning, somewhat simple people with very clear-cut Fundamentalist ideas of right and wrong. Although the patient had rebelled considerably against her parents' religious beliefs during adolescence, she and her family had remained on good terms and quite close. She had been her father's favorite, had felt closer to him than to her mother, and they had shared many intellectual . interests. She had repeated many aspects of her relationship with her father in the relationship with the minister, and subsequently repeated these early in treatment with me. She felt that she and her mother had never had very much in common and described her mother as timid, overanxious, and not much interested in anything outside of the home. This was in contrast to the patient, who, although very interested in her husband and children, read a great deal and was active in local politics. The patient felt that her mother had been much less helpful than she might have been during her growing up. This particularly referred to adolescence when the patient had been quite rebellious and argumentative in her attempts to free herself from this somewhat close and restrictive family. The patient's mother had handled her rebellion by silent but visible worry and by impatiently telling the patient that she had to learn to think for herself. The patient felt let down by her mother's refusal to help. These were, of course, current complaints as well. This problem recurred in treatment in that she was very anxious about allowing herself any regression with me at first and felt that I, too, placed a high premium on her acting like an adult no matter how she felt.

Her childhood had been relatively unproblematic. She had done well in school, had had a series of best friends, been popular in high school, had begun to date then and had been "in love" with two different men before she met and married her husband. In late high school and college she had vague career plans of teaching English literature and of writing. She did teach for a while early in her marriage while her husband was still in school, and she had continued to write poetry for her own pleasure until the birth of their first child. She began again to write poetry in the months following the appearance of the metastases.

Her husband was a warm, sensitive, intelligent, ambitious young man who shared his life with her to her very great pleasure. Except for occasional arguments about his somewhat problematic and widowed mother who periodically decided she wanted to come to live with them, the marriage had presented no problems. Mrs. B. was basically a cheerful, optimistic, highly intelligent woman who had derived much pleasure from her marriage and her children. Her sexual life had been deeply satisfying to her and another contributing factor to her presenting depression was that pain and fatigue, combined with some reluctance on her husband's part, had sharply decreased the frequency of sexual intercourse in the months preceding my seeing her. She attributed falling in love with the minister to this. She was very worried that her husband no longer found her attractive now that she was ill.

The patient's relationships to her two sons were complex. Both were happy, spontaneous boys whom she enjoyed. It early became apparent that she at times identified with the older boy. As she became less and less well and more concerned about dying, she became fearful about his starting school without her and about how lonely she expected he might feel. A major goal for her became that she stay alive until he was safely started in school and not "by himself." In fact, she did accomplish this, became totally bed-ridden shortly after he started school, and died within three weeks. She had much less to say about her younger son. It was apparent that this relationship had been considerably more ambivalent from the start because the malignancy had been part of the pregnancy and the early months of his life. She struggled to fight off the irrational feeling that she might never have had cancer had it not been for this pregnancy. It felt to her increasingly that he was living at her expense and she was much troubled by her impatience with him. Talking about this helped substantially, but their relationship was never free from problems. It was this son about whom she most worried during a brief period in which she wondered if cancer might be either hereditary or contagious.

Treatment can perhaps most easily be summarized in terms of her relationship to me. The very fact of her prospective death had seriously disturbed her relationships with those who meant most to her but had in no way impaired her need for people, had in fact increased it. She very quickly became intensely involved with me. My statement that she was entitled to help and comfort and my intervention regarding the drugs undoubtedly facilitated this. In the second hour she questioned me about my training and my professional life and made it clear that she was worried that I might feel as defeated about her dying as her other doctors seemed to. I assured her that I was willing to help her in any way that I could and that this certainly included helping her with her feelings about dying. When she asked if this might not make me uncomfortable, I replied that I would try to help her in any event. She then began to discuss religion and philosophy with me, in large part I think to see whether I was really willing to help her with her feelings or would, like her parents and the minister, succumb to religious platitudes or withdraw out of my own discomfort. I did neither, and out of these discussions emerged several problems. She was afraid of dying alone, of becoming less and less attractive, "sick," and having people lose interest in her, a fear which was partially substantiated by the way her family had turned away from her. She also feared the gradually increasing sense of helplessness that her physical incapacitation was giving rise to and was in part using her intelligence to help to master this difficult situation. She was also using the philosophic discussions in an attempt to gain my approval of how "adult" she was being. Discussion of these problems gradually led to a diminution of her depression, complete absence of any talk of suicide, impressive absence of anxiety, and an increased sense of well-being and of hope which was quite at odds with her deteriorating physical condition. She was physically more comfortable during this period because of adequate medication. At this same time she asked to borrow some books of mine, which I loaned her, and she began to bring me poetry which she had written earlier. I quote one poem to illustrate her preoccupation with separation.

To die is such a lonely thing,
We cannot take one friend along.
To hold a hand would make it
Far less a frightening song.

With this she began to share with me her grief over dying, which to her essentially meant leaving those she loved best. Despite occasional interruptions by her worsening physical condition, mourning continued in one form or another until her final coma. She began by talking about the relationship to the minister and how hurt and angry she had been at his misunderstanding her need for him and his present avoidance of her. She told me in detail how they had met, the discussions they had had about her illness, and what they discussed during the times she was discouraged. She wept over his leaving her when she needed him most. She was very scornful of this kind of "religion," but also felt that he was to be pitied as he apparently did not have the strength to remain with her to help.

This led to her feelings about her husband's withdrawing from her. She understood that he was grieving himself, was hurt by his inability to help her with her feelings, but for the most part was protective about his feelings. Except for occasionally talking of feeling irritated by the lengthy hours he worked, she expressed little anger about him. She gradually told me about her marriage and relationship to her husband, of their courtship, honeymoon, the earlier happy times that they had had, his hopes and aspirations about his profession, and how she shared these. She was deeply grieved by the fact that she would not be around to continue to share his life with him; she hoped he would marry again, but preferred not to think about this. She discussed both pregnancies and her relationships with both sons in equal detail, again with emphasis on how sorely she would miss future participation in their lives. She allowed herself some daydreaming as to what she hoped their futures would be like. All of this seemed very much like working through in mourning, was accompanied by appropriate crying and by occasional denial, although the denial was almost always in the form of giving herself an extra year or so of life, not of being cured. Her ego never permitted her any convincing fantasies of a hereafter in which she might continue to be aware of the lives of those she loved. Death to her meant the end of these relationships and a separation from those she loved best. She was angry at the unfairness of her early death and talked with intense feeling of the impending loss of those she loved most and the experiences she would never have with them. She tried to console herself by reminding herself of the things she had already had, but until she was much sicker physically, she found little comfort in this.

She was both angry about and defeated by her parents' current minimal participation in her life. For the most part, however, she viewed her parents protectively and felt she was saving them pain by not insisting they spend time with her. This seemed to repeat aspects of her adolescent emancipation from her parents. Memories of earlier aspects of her relationship to them never appeared directly except for the nostalgia for the intellectual relationship she had shared with her father, which was now precluded by his age and illness as well as by his feelings about her death.

Her pain and insomnia during this six-week period were well controlled by drugs, but her weakness and weight loss were increasing, and she had had several hemorrhages from minor bruises. Her surgeon decided to hospitalize her for another course of X ray and for transfusions. By this time she was beginning to look grotesque because of skull metastases, and shortly after hospitalization she became comatose, presumably from increased intracranial pressure. She was promptly treated and regained consciousness gradually over a period of three days.

First Regression: Externalization of
Superego and Identification

However, this sudden severe clinical change brought about a striking change in our relationship, the first obvious regression, and from this point on there was no question that she was repeating with me aspects of her earlier relationship with her mother. She herself perceived the regression and was briefly apologetic "for being such a baby," but as I explained this as an expected part of her illness, she became less ashamed. My manifest response to her underwent a change at this time, too, in that she was obviously much sicker, and communication was no longer on an exclusively verbal level. She frequently needed physical care during the time

I spent with her, and I made her bed comfortable, fed her at times, and at other times simply sat quietly with her. She often asked me to stay with her while she fell asleep. Essentially I responded to her regression by assuming certain necessary kinds of ego functions for her, in effect began to function as an external ego in much the same sense that the mother's ego functions as an external ego for that of the developing child. Clinically, the patient's affective response made it easily possible to judge the amount of this that was necessary: too little help made her ashamed about the regression, whereas too much made her impatient and angry with me.

As she became more alert, she reported the only dreams she told me during therapy. These were a series of dream fragments having to do with physical activity: she was a child again and running happily; she was swimming at the country club to which she belonged; she was jumping rope as a young girl; she was playing tennis as she had done the previous summer. All of these dreams seemed essentially to represent the wish to be well and active; they also illustrate regression to the simple wish-fulfillment dreams of childhood. They were reported with sadness, but, as she associated to them, she began to be irritated with me. Discussion of the irritation brought into focus her intense envy of me, which had been present but unverbalized from the beginning. She envied my relative youth, my health, my activity, the fact that I was not sick and helpless as she was. She also was jealous of me, said she had recently become very troubled by a recurring idea that I might marry her husband and care for her children after her death. She also reported that she was even more worried that her mother-in-law would replace her with her children and had made her husband promise that he would not permit his mother to move in with him after her death. Her jealousy and envy of the minister's wife had also been intense, but she had been too ashamed of this to tell me earlier. As she spoke of these feelings about me she first apologized but gradually became very angry and demanded that I stop seeing her because the comparison between our relative states of health and attractiveness was more than she could bear. I told her that these feelings were certainly understandable in these circumstances, that I understood how angry she was at me, but that I did not feel that this precluded our continuing to work together, that I really wanted to help her. I also made the only transference interpretation I ever made to her, vague and incomplete though it was: that part of what troubled her was that because she was sick, she was refeeling with me some of the feelings she had had as a child about being a child and not able to do what her mother did. She seemed relieved by this, smiled, and said she had changed her mind about firing me. Both of these issues came up several times again but never with the same intensity, and were more often apparent in attempts to identify with me. She knew my schedule of teaching activities, for instance, and would imagine herself in my role at various times of the day, spent considerable time imagining what I was doing and where I was. The oedipal transference was readily apparent and the ambivalence apparently solved by her childlike identification with the positive side of the ambivalence. In essence I allowed her to externalize her punitive superego and gave her an ego ideal she could live up to when I accepted the jealousy and envy as part of her illness.

Her strength partially returned and she again went home and resumed some care of the children. The older boy's starting school increasingly became a focus of worry and, for her, a compelling reason to husband her energies. She made repeated references to the hope he would not have to do this without her as she was sure this would be terrifying for him. Initially this was a puzzling preoccupation, especially so in that her own first days at school had not been in any way disturbing, a fact confirmed by the patient's mother as well as by the patient. Continued discussion of this, however, indicated that she was equating his starting school with her own approaching death and that she was quite troubled by the idea that she "knew no one there," would in effect be a stranger among strangers as she expected her son to feel in his early days at school. That this patient had had no deaths in those closest to her may have contributed to this preoccupation as she had no one to "join in death" in fantasy (Brodsky, 1954; Jones, 1911).

After a brief period at home, she again became so weak that hospitalization was necessary for rest and for transfusions. She had been complaining of periodic visual difficulties for several weeks and feared she was losing her sight, although she had hopefully attributed this to bouts of weakness. While in the hospital she gradually became intermittently blind. She showed more severe anxiety about this than she had about any previous symptom. It was a concrete sign of the nearness of her death, of course, but to her this meant that she was about to be completely cut off from the people around her, by this time especially from me, and she was terrified of what she envisioned as a life in which she was mentally alert but remote from contact with people.

Second Regression: Externalization of Ego

During the first few days of her blindness I spent extra time with her and at her request visually described and identified for her hospital personnel and the details of her room; she was particularly interested in knowing what clothing I was wearing and was pleased when it was something familiar to her. I also did my utmost to demonstrate that, while visual communication was seriously interfered with, we retained the equally important avenues of communication of talking and of touch. She likened these to the way a baby must feel, that feeling physical closeness and hearing the sound of mother's voice might be of as basic importance as seeing. I read to her—she particularly liked the 23rd and 121st Psalms—and I sat close enough that she could touch me or I, her at any time. She often drowsed or fell asleep during these hours, and I had the impression that my physical presence and the tone of my voice were almost more important than the verbal content of what I said.

This outbreak of acute anxiety, in fact the only such outbreak during treatment, at a time when her relationship to me was threatened by blindness is an impressive illustration of the level of ego regression. By this time I had assumed for her many aspects of ego functioning. Her anxiety signaled the danger of ego disruption at the threatened loss of my supporting ego. This is, of course, an infantile form of separation anxiety. I responded to her anxiety with a marked increase in my availability to her and by "loaning" her my sight as well as by reassuring her that her loss of sight did not mean a disruption of our relationship. Her anxiety diminished with this.

Third Regression: Introjection

Further ego regression assured continuation of the relationship, for soon thereafter she began to talk of an all-pervasive sense of peace and contentment which was quite at odds with the clinical picture but was related to what she described as her "silly illogical imagination." Instead of imagining me in the various aspects of my life, she now felt I was with her twenty-four hours a day and she began to carry on imaginary conversations with me. Most of these that she reported at this time dealt with discussions of her feelings, but increasingly she felt as if I were always there comforting her, assuaging pain or physical discomfort and telling her she need not be afraid, that she was not alone.

She felt that her death was quickly approaching, asked that she be allowed to die at home, and I encouraged her sister to come and care for her there. At home she rallied briefly to get her older son started in school and then became partially bedridden. Her sister cared for her physical needs, and we both continued to talk with her, read to her, and to keep her as comfortable as we could. She drowsed frequently but remained very much alert and interested in the lives of her family when she was awake. The blindness was intermittent during these weeks. She began occasionally to call her sister by my first name and at the same time to me made several uncorrected slips of calling me "mother" (Saul, 1959). She questioned me closely about the time of my last visit and the length of my current visit (I was seeing her twice a day at this point) and always expressed surprise at my answers as she now "almost" had the conviction that I was always there. Occasionally she would wake in pain and be surprised to find me absent.

Eissler, in *The Psychiatrist and the Dying Patient,* says, "It is conceivable that through the establishment of transference, through an approach which mobilizes the archaic trust in the world and reawakens the primordial feelings of being protected by a mother, the suffering of the dying can be reduced to a minimum even in case of extreme physical pain" (1955). Freud also mentions this as a possibility (1926). The psychological suffering of the patient is also reduced to a minimum; in fact, this sense of peace and contentment seemed massively to protect against all affects of unpleasure. It was only at times of severe physical pain that the protection of this "hallucination" failed and then only briefly and without anixety; the expectation was that I would "soon" arrive and provide relief. Here the regressive level is to that developmental stage in which the object is clearly perceived as an object, felt as continuously present, and the borders between external and internal are at times hazy. This not only had the effect of minimizing physical pain and psychological suffering but also seemed to prevent the narcissistic, hypochondriacal preoccupation that is so frequently a part of serious illness. That this level of regression in object relations coexisted with nonregressed ego functioning in other areas indicates only the complexity of the concept of regression.

She remained troubled by the conflict between this feeling of my continuous presence and the reality of the situation, however, and began to talk of her unhappiness that I would not be with her when she died. I at first thought she was referring to my physical presence and tried to reassure her, but it turned out that she had long since taken my presence during her death as an established fact. What she meant was that I would not be dying with her, that this we could not share.

Three days before her death and a few hours before she became terminally comatose, we had a long conversation about her dying. She told me her only remaining fear was that dying was strange and unknown to her, that she had never done it before. Like birth, it was something that only happened once to any individual, and that similarly one might not remember what it was really like, only know that it had once happened. She no longer worried about what was to happen to her after death any more than an infant being born could worry about what his future life might be; she felt that she might be unnecessarily concerned with the actual process of death itself. She then asked me if I had been with other patients when they died and seemed relieved by my affirmative answer. One very comforting recurring thought to her was that throughout the centuries many people had died before her; more importantly, it had occurred to her that I would share this experience with her, although not at this time. I agreed that this was certainly so and added that I hoped I might equal her courage. She was pleased by this, and she then reminisced about our relationship. She recalled our first meeting and smiled in retrospect at her needless reluctance at seeing a psychiatrist. She thanked me for having helped her, particularly not to commit suicide, which she now felt would have been most difficult for her family, especially her sons. I was obviously moved by the finality of all this, and she chided me about being much more involved with her than doctors should be with their patients, and abruptly cried. Her regret was that we had known each other so briefly, that she was dying without ever knowing me really well. I said she had known me rather better than she might think, that I felt it a great privilege that she had shared this experience with me and that I, too, wished we had had more time together. She asked me if after her death I would wear for her a red dress she had bought just before she became too sick to have any fun—she wanted "the dress to have some fun." I agreed, thanked her, asked whether there was anything else I might do for her, and she asked that I again read the 23rd Psalm. In the midst of this she interrupted me by crying. She said she would miss me terribly but somehow knew I was "always there" and asked that I hold her hand while she fell asleep. I did, and this was the last time the patient was conscious except for very brief periods that afternoon. She became comatose later on in the day and died three days later without regaining consciousness.

Eissler feels that mourning would ease the plight of the dying patient by accomplishing a decathexis of objects prior to death and that therefore death could be accepted as a "natural consequence of an energic constellation in that moment." But he feels that this is not likely while "perception conveys the fact of the existence of the love objects" (1955). Mourning was a very prominent feature of this patient's last few months of life; although part of this seemed to have resulted from the emotional withdrawal of those around her, part was also related to her knowledge of her death, its meaning to her of separation, and to the physical changes in herself. It is worth noting that the order in which she grieved was chronologically significant. She began with the most recent relationship, the minister, and followed this by mourning the loss of her husband, and her parents. The grief about her two sons was a relatively continuous process in that mourning them was very intimately related to mourning the loss of her health, her productivity, and her own future. What seemed to happen was that libido detached from objects through mourning gradually found a transference substitute in me. However, at the end she was presented with the impending conclusion of our relationship by her death. During the last hour she mourned this but also solved the problem by extending her own life through me through the gift of the red dress, and by taking me with her in death "although not at this time."

Discussion

This case has been presented in considerable detail because of the relative rarity of such cases in the literature and because of its theoretical and therapeutic implications. The patient's presenting despair and grief about dying are far from unusual; that family, friends, physicians, and clergy often turn from the dying in one way or another need not surprise us. As Eissler points out, many factors have tended to exclude the psychiatrist or the analyst from the bedside of the dying patient, not the least of which are the unusual demands on time (1955).

Eissler says that the technique of the treatment of the dying patient must center around what he calls "the gift situation" in which the psychiatrist must create the proper time to make the right gift. The gift is experienced by the patient as "an unusual . . . favor of destiny." This case would suggest that the really crucial gift the therapist can give is that of himself as an available object. The treatment of this patient can be simply summarized as a process in which I helped the patient to defend herself against object loss by facilitating the development of a regressive relationship to me which precluded object loss.

The patient came into treatment with me anxious, depressed, and contemplating suicide in her despair over the failure of those around her to respond to her need for them. Once she established my willingness to be with her and to try to help, she quickly agreed to psychiatric treatment. She initially tested my willingness to help her by engaging me in religious and philosophic discussions of the meaning of death, as if to make certain that I would not be driven away by the mention of death as an abstraction. In retrospect, I think she was also exploring my own attitudes about death. Satisfied that I could listen and remain with her, she then allowed herself to grieve with me the actual and potential losses she was facing—her husband, children, family, her health, and her future.

While the mourning was still in progress, she became temporarily physically very ill, briefly comatose, and from this point on she was consciously very preoccupied with her relationship to me.

One of her first worries on regaining consciousness and perceiving her regression was that she might have become "too much of a baby" for me to continue to help. When I reassured her about this, she for the first time began to express the envious, hostile competitiveness of the oedipal transference, which was also a threat to the relationship. My interpretation of this combined with her intense need for a relatively unambivalent relationship with me allowed her to reexternalize her superego and to identify with the positive side of the oedipal ambivalence.

Later on, when blindness intervened, the anxiety was again that this seriously threatened her relationship to me. She solved this by a further regression to a level of object relationship in which she hallucinated my presence and the boundaries of external and internal were at times blurred. The tenacity with which she clung to this object relationship despite all vicissitudes was extremely impressive. In the last hour she solved the problem of threatened loss of me by feeling that I would be with her in death, "although not at this time." In the course of dying this patient's ego permitted massive regression in many areas, all of which was apparently in the service of maintaining an intensely cathected object relationship with me.

The protection this relationship provided her against anxiety and depression was extremely impressive. Although she grieved throughout treatment, depression was never a serious problem, and the only massive anxiety occurred briefly at the time of her blindness. In addition, despite both pulmonary and bone metastases, she was relatively free from pain on comparatively small amounts of morphine. Freud remarks in *Inhibitions, Symptoms and Anxiety* that "when there is a psychical diversion brought about by some other interest, even the most intense physical pains fail to arise" (1926). This case amply bears this out. Interestingly enough, the intensity of the relationship also precluded the increased narcissism and bodily preoccupation that are so frequently associated with severe illness. It would certainly suggest that such symptoms, often assumed to be an inevitable part of the chronic or fatal illness, can be obviated by a therapeutic approach such as the one presented here. It is tempting to speculate that at least in certain patients many problems frequently met with in dying patients, i.e., denial, anxiety, depression, increased narcissism and apathy, may be a result of actual or anticipated object loss and are by no means intrinsic to the psychological response to death. Certainly there is no question that a therapeutic approach such as I have outlined could be expected substantially to ease the suffering of many dying patients and add greatly to our knowledge of the metapsychology of dying.

In summary, the essential therapeutic tools in the treatment of the dying patient are the therapist's constant availability as an object, his reliability, his empathy, and his ability to respond appropriately to the patient's needs. Once Mrs. B. was truly convinced I meant it when I said I would be with her until her death, she made few demands for extra time; I did, however, offer this unasked at crucial times for her, such as during the early days of her blindness.

An essential prerequisite of therapy with the dying is consciously accepted countertransference. The dying patient specifically confronts the analyst with guilt and with an injury to his narcissism; that the patient is actually dying inevitably mobilizes the analyst's childhood death wishes and at the same time serves as a painful reminder of his own mortality. Defenses against either or both countertransferences in large part explain why dying patients are so often left to die alone. The analyst's defenses against these will distance him from the patient in one way or another and inevitably seriously interfere with his ability to respond appropriately to the patient's needs. The last hour illustrates this well. Both the patient and I knew she was very close to death; she solved the problem of our separation by taking me with her in death. She generously provided me with a partial defense by adding "although not at this time." She also relinquished to me the oedipal struggle by bequeathing me her favorite dress, the one she had bought "for fun." I was aware of grief, guilt, anxiety, and anger during this hour, but I am sure it is apparent that defenses against any of these countertransference responses, whether denial, reassurance, repression, overprotectiveness, false optimism, or intellectualization, would have markedly interfered with my usefulness to the patient as the object she needed. My conscious awareness of the sources of these responses was what made it possible for me to respond appropriately in terms of her needs. In essence, the dying patient inevitably provokes countertransference responses in the analyst, but acceptance and utilization of these can be most therapeutic for the patient.

Summary

A case report of the treatment of a patient during the last three and a half months of her life has been presented. The case suggests that a major psychological problem of the dying patient is that of both actual and threatened object loss. A method of treatment has been described which provides massive protection against both physical pain and psychological unpleasure, and certain theoretical conclusions about the psychological problems of the dying have been drawn.

BIBLIOGRAPHY

ARONSEN, G. J. (1959). "Treatment of the Dying Person." In: *The Meaning of Death,* ed. H. Feifel. New York: McGraw-Hill, pp. 251–258.

BRODSKY, B. (1959). "Liebestod Fantasies in a Patient Faced with a Fatal Illness." *Int. J. Psa.,* XL.

EISSLER, K. R. (1955). *The Psychiatrist and the Dying Patient.* New York: International Universities Press.

FEIFEL, H. (1959). "Attitudes Toward Death in Some Normal and Mentally Ill Populations." In: *The Meaning of Death,* ed. H. Feifel. New York: McGraw-Hill, pp. 114–130.

FREUD, S. (1915) . *Thoughts for the Times on War and Death.* Standard Edition, XIV. London: Hogarth Press, 1957.

———— (1916). *On Transcience.* Standard Edition, XIV. London: Hogarth Press, 1957.

————(1926). *Inhibitions, Symptoms and Anxiety.* Standard Edition, XX. London: Hogarth Press, 1959.

JONES, E. (1911). "Dying Together." *Essays in Applied Psychoanalysis,* I. London: Hogarth Press, 1951.

LESHAN, L. & LESHAN, E. (1951) . "Psychotherapy in the Patient with a Limited Life-Span." *Psychiatry,* XXIV.

SANDFORD, B. (1957). "Some Notes on a Dying Patient." *Int. J. Psa.* XXXVIII.

SAUL L. (1959). "Reactions of a Man to Natural Death." *Psa. Quart.,* XXVIII.

WEISMAN, A. B. & HACKETT, T. P. (1961). "Predilection to Death." *Psychosom. Med.,* XXIII.

III. ON THE "LONGING TO DIE"

KATE FRIEDLANDER

Considering that attempts at suicide are not uncommon during analysis and that they represent a very serious complication, it is rather astonishing that the literature on the subject is not more extensive. I am therefore venturing in the present paper to describe the suicidal mechanism of a single case. I do this only because I am of the opinion that this particular mechanism is not uncommon and often actually results in suicide.

In psychoanalytical literature we find at least two ways of approach to the problem of suicide.

The one, which I shall do no more than mention as it has no actual bearing on the problem which I want to discuss here, is the psychoanalytical interpretation of statistics (19), taking into account different cultures and different circumstances. We know that in certain cultures suicide is considered to be a respectable act and that therefore suicide is not necessarily a sign of illness and we also know that in certain circumstances the number of suicides may suddenly increase and include otherwise healthy people. These considerations have not necessarily any bearing on the mechanism of the suicidal act. The fact that in certain circumstances normal people may commit suicide does not exclude the possibility that under these special conditions mechanisms come into play which in normal circumstances are only to be found in neurotic people.

In order to find out what particular mechanism is involved one has to study the mechanism in any given case, and this is the second way of approach to the problem.

The question which I want to examine is whether the melancholic type of suicide is the basis for every suicide committed or whether there are cases or perhaps a whole group of cases in which other mechanisms are the basis for suicide or attempts at suicide.

Before the publication of "Mourning and Melancholia" (7) it was assumed that various libidinal impulses may lead to suicide. Ernest Jones (14, 15) emphasized that, apart from coprophilic, sadistic and incestuous tendencies, certain libidinal fantasies, concerning for instance the anal conception of childbirth, may be acted out in the love-condition of dying together. Jones furthermore expressed the opinion that "the idea of personal death does not exist for the unconscious, being always replaced by that of sexual communion or of birth." The question of suicide was also discussed in Vienna in 1910 (25, 5). Various libidinal factors, such as disappointment in love, feelings of guilt, a desire to be punished or revenge, were stated to lead to suicide. Sadger (20) expressed the current opinion very well when he said: "Nobody will kill himself who has not entirely given up the hope of being loved." Freud (9) ended the discussion by stating that the main problem had not been solved, namely, what makes it possible for the very strong impulse of self-preservation to be overcome. He was then in doubt whether libidinal disappointment alone would be sufficient to overcome the instinct to live or whether the ego can resign itself out of ego-motives. Freud (7) solved the question two years later in his paper "Mourning and Melancholia." The melancholiac who either in reality or in fantasy has suffered the loss of a beloved object is unable to free his libido from the object and its associations. Owing to the prevalent type of narcissistic object-choice, the lost object of the melancholiac becomes introjected. Furthermore, in melancholia regression has taken place to the oral-sadistic phase, so that ambivalence, and with it sadism, are pronounced. The aggression directed against the original object becomes directed against the individual's self or rather against the introjected object. Owing to the severity of the super-ego, in which destructive impulses are prevalent, the patient is forced to destroy himself.

This explanation solved a number of hitherto obscure problems and for years no further advance was made beyond confirmation of the validity of this mode of suicide. Apparently until recently it was assumed that every suicidal act, whether it happens in a melancholic or in a neurotic case, even in hysteria, is based on the same mechanism of aggressions directed against the individual's self and the prevalence of destructive impulses over libidinal ones (2, 3, 4, 13, 17).

In recent years the question has sometimes arisen whether mechanisms other than the melancholic ones may also be responsible for certain types of suicide. Garma (12) stresses the importance of the variable significance of the conception of death in suicide and gives a very valuable scheme in which the libidinal factors involved in suicide are clearly shown. M. Schmideberg (21) emphasizes the importance of libidinal factors and maintains that it is very often "not the 'death instinct' which drives a person to suicide, but strong emotional disturbances—especially anxiety—which interfere with the self-preserving instinct." It is not quite clear to me whether she believes that in a melancholic case there is also no genuine wish for death, or whether she means that suicidal mechanisms can be different in different cases. No attempt is made to classify the mechanisms in different cases but the various libidinal impulses which may drive to suicide or to substitutes for suicide are explained.

Zilboorg (24) doubts wheher all motivations for suicide are to be explained by the classical formula and describes one mechanism which seems to him to be different and for which he finds parallels in the rites of primitive people: namely, the compulsion to become identified with a dead person who has died before the mechanism of identification is completed. Zilboorg's idea is apparently that, apart from the classical melancholic type of suicide, there is at least this other type in which the active impulse to die is based on a libidinal impulse.

A clinical classification of suicidal cases has been attempted by Federn (5, 6), who points out that there are two groups of abnormal characters found in patients who attempt or commit suicide: people who are inclined to be depressed and people with an inclination to be addicts. To these two groups belong hysterical, obsessional neurotic and neurasthenic patients or even people with no outspoken neurosis at all. To the group of the addicts belong not only really addicted people, but all people who react in the same particular way. The immediate reaction to a frustration is with this type of person an increase of tension until the tension is unbearable. The addict thinks that it is better to die than to go without the thing for which he craves. The suffering is not fictitious but real; it leads to an increased want and death seems to be pleasurable in relieving the unbearable tension. The depression of these people is not as deep as in melancholiacs, but this type is less able to stand tension and suffering which the melancholiac at least partly enjoys. Federn (6) states that the melancholiac has to suffer from that which he has lost, whilst the addict has to suffer for that which he cannot get. Federn's idea apparently is that the reason for suicide is different in these two groups, but it is not clear to me whether he means that the suicidal mechanism is in both groups aggression directed against the individual's self. It seems to me that there is a decisive difference between the mechanisms of the two groups: the addict type wants to die because that seems to him to be more pleasurable than to stand the tension; death is desired in accordance with the pleasure principle.

The case I am going to take has some resemblance to what Federn describes as the addict type. I want to prove that the mechanism which eventually led to the attempts at suicide was due to libidinal impulses.

The patient is a man of twenty-nine years of age in good external circumstances. During the time when the attempts at suicide happened no disturbing external event took place and the patient did not try to give rationalizations in the form of external circumstances as reason for his attempts. He has a masochistic character. The conscious conflict which drives him to attempt suicide is the following. He has a brother who is eight years his senior, and of whom he is jealous: his brother has had so many girls, probably about 200, whilst he, the patient, cannot even get one. His mother therefore respects the elder brother much more than him. He believes that his mother has the same attitude toward him as his brother has: namely, that for him it is not necessary to have a girl. It therefore does not help him just to find a girl, because his brother and his mother would only sneer at him and find the girl not attractive enough. He therefore prefers to stay ill and have no girl at all than to be healthy and be satisfied with a girl who would be inferior to his brother's friends. As he cannot get a girl, he wants to die.

I must point out that behind the oedipus situation which expresses itself in this conflict lies an oral fixation caused by oral cravings and an oral disappointment in his mother. Hatred against mother and brother are openly expressed with fantasies about their death without any conscious feeling of guilt. The feeling of guilt is compensated by oral and anal frustrations which the patient imposes upon himself. He is extremely ascetic in his food, although he can experience pleasure from eating, and he does not allow himself to spend a penny on pleasurable things. But he gives comparatively large sums of money to a charity which, interestingly enough, is for buying milk for poor children.

His sexual activities are somewhat limited. He has masturbated since he was fourteen, at times with homosexual and beating fantasies. Occasionally he visits prostitutes.

His first attempt at suicide was, as he called it himself, a staging of a suicide. He closed the windows and door of his room and turned on the gas stove. He had heard that on breathing in gas one becomes drowsy and sleepy, and he intended to go on until he became drowsy and then wanted to stop it. The smell of the gas was noticed by his landlady and he had to interrupt his performance.

Some time later he began to be interested in veronal, as he had heard that it was a drug which could induce sleep without bad after-effects. He studied the action and dosage of the drug carefully from books on pharmacology. He then bought a large amount of it in France, where he could get it cheap and without a prescription. He had read that 40–50 grs., that is 3–4 grm., was the lethal dose. One day he took 28 grs., that is 2 grm., in broad daylight when he was sitting in the park. He did not feel any effect from it. He then took 36 grs., that is 2.5 grm., a little less than what he considered to be the lethal dose. He slept for two days without interruption and felt the after-effects for nearly a week. Some months later he again took 36 grs., that is 2.5 grm., in two doses each of six tablets. Apart from these two serious attempts, he twice took 18 grs., that is, 1.3 grm., in order to sleep over the weekend. Ordinarily he never takes any drugs at all.

The occasions on which he attempted suicide were very similar. The first attempt happened one weekend; the two serious attempts happened at Christmas and at Easter when he would not be coming to analysis for four days. At the same time his brother was away, once on a visit to his mother, who lives twelve hours' distance away, and once on a visit to a couple, where the wife was interested in his brother and the patient was slightly interested in her, too. On other occasions, when the brother was away on business or I was away on holidays, he did not make any attempt and the thought of suicide did not occur to him.

The psychic situation which induces the patient to make the attempt is in every case the same. Consciously he cannot bear the thought of the time which is in front of him, each time four days, without a girl. The thought of the brother makes him furious and the only way out seems to be for him to go to sleep. He desires to sleep for four days without interruption. He has no conscious thought then that he wants to end his life by taking the drug and actually takes a little less than what is considered to be the lethal dose. He has a vague idea that afterwards everything will be perfectly all right. He has no anxiety and no doubt as to how the drug is going to act. Everything is engulfed in the craving for the drug which will make him sleep and in dwelling on how pleasurable that will be.

Analysis reveals the various mechanisms involved in this attempt at suicide:

(1) By killing himself he can take revenge on his brother, his mother and his analyst. His brother will feel guilty because he has left him alone. His mother, who in reality only cares for his bodily welfare and not for his happiness, will be terribly upset about his death. He can prove by his death to what it is that analysis really leads.

(2) He is able to satisfy his intense oral craving only if it results in death, that is, if he pays for it with his death. The mode of his attempts, namely that he takes drugs, is here significant. His description of his longing to take the drug in this particular situation is very similar to that of an addict.

(3) The act is also a fantasy that by going to sleep he becomes united with his brother as well as with his mother. Probably this union occurs by way of introjection, as various fantasies seem to prove.

(4) When he was very small, probably under two years of age, he used sometimes to cry helplessly for his mother to come back, until he fell asleep. When he woke up, his mother was there. This fantasy also shows clearly that what he really wants is not to die but to sleep in order to find his mother when he wakes up again. That is

why it is so important to him to take a large amount of the drug and not simply two tablets morning and night. He does not wish to wake up at all during the four days before he can come to analysis again.

(5) There are various fantasies which show that he has great pleasure in imagining what his brother and mother will say when he is dead. Then they will appreciate how much he has suffered and how badly they have treated him. It is significant that at that time he did not want to have a certain amount of money in his name. In case he should commit suicide he does not want his brother and his mother to pay death duties and for that reason to be sorry about his death. He wants to be mourned because mother and brother loved him for that reason only.

To sum up, the factors involved in this suicidal mechanism are revenge, satisfaction of his strong oral desires, and the fantasy of being saved by his loving mother. As a fantasy, these factors, which are without doubt derived from libidinal impulses only, are by no means rare; on the contrary these elements or some of them, such as taking revenge or the wish to be saved from a dangerous situation, are most common. But patients who very often express such suicidal fantasies may never actually attempt suicide, especially if they become conscious of their libidinal wishes.

The question which has to be solved is, therefore: What special forces are working in this case so that the fantasy is acted out in this dangerous way? In trying to solve the problem which I raised at the beginning, we have to ask the question: Are the forces which drive the man to commit suicide derived from destructive impulses?—which means: Are they aggressions directed against his own self? Does he really want to kill introjected objects or is another mechanism at work?

The patient's aggressions are openly directed against his real love objects, his brother and his mother, and are expressed in many ways. As I have mentioned before, his feelings of guilt are compensated in such a way that he is able to express his hatred against his love objects in fantasy as well as in reality. The patient has no inclination to reproach himself and he does not do so; he does not believe himself to be inferior and therefore not worthy to live. In his moods of depression he reproaches the world and especially his love objects and is waiting for them to give him what he wants.

The patient is entirely fixated to his infantile objects, but not only in fantasy. His only real object-relations today are those with his relatives, his brother and his mother. Of course, both of them have infantile traces and he does not see them as they really are. But it is not only the infantile imago of these people that exists in him; on the contrary, he is still attracted to the living persons. It is significant that he can only have a sexual relationship if his brother and mother are in another town, the further away the better. Apparently he is then able to shift some of his object libido on to other objects.

Furthermore, I think it is clear that the patient's ultimate aim is not to destroy himself. He merely wants to sleep in order to wake up to a better life in which all his wishes are fulfilled. Nor does he want to destroy his brother and his mother, since before his attempt at suicide these objects are not introjected, but exist for him in the outside world. In the act of taking in the drug he introjects his beloved objects, but this introjection serves a libidinal aim, namely, union with his mother and not her destruction. Here we see some resemblance between this mechanism and the mechanism of the ecstatic suicide, in which the aim is to be united with the dead lover or with God.

So it seems to be that the force which drives the patient to act out his fantasy is not derived from destructive impulses. To express it in a simpler way, the patient does not want to destroy himself. Actually his attempts at suicide are very pleasurable and when he comes to his analyst after such an attempt he is elated, like somebody who has achieved what he wants and not as if he has failed. If he really wanted to die he would have failed in his purpose.

Nevertheless his attempts are very serious and self-destruction might easily be the result. The astonishing fact is that, although the patient clearly does not want to die, he makes his attempts in a rather dangerous way. He takes a large amount of the drug, which might kill him, especially as he is living alone and might stay in his room for days without being missed.

The question arises why the patient does not take more precautions against dying if it is true that he does not want his attempt to succeed. And now we see the interesting fact that he does take precautions but that these precautions are not sufficient. He takes a little less than the lethal dose. If the lethal dose is 40 grs., he takes 36 grs. He leaves the window open because his mother told him once that fresh air is healthy. When he wakes up after two days he rings up either myself or his medical practitioner. These precautions seem to be and really are childish and incompatible with the high intelligence of the patient. But this strange behavior becomes clearer if one is aware of the fact that somehow the patient has a conviction that whatever he does his mother is sure to save him. This conviction is so strong that it severely disturbs his sense of reality, and this disturbance of his sense of reality is the one factor which lets the patient act out his fantasy in such a dangerous way. Instead of facing reality, he still has an infantile belief in the omnipotence of his parents. The important thing is not what he himself does but what he expects to be his mother's wish.

With this consideration, the mechanism of his attempt at suicide becomes clearer; what we see here is a *"Kinderselbstmord,"* the attempt at suicide of a child. In the suicidal fantasies of children the same libidinal factors are at work as we have seen in this case. If we take as an example the suicidal fantasy of Tom Sawyer which was described analytically by Schneider (22), we see that Tom and his friends want to die because they have experienced a disappointment in love. They want to take revenge and are very much interested in the mourning of the grown-ups, who will at last understand what good boys they are. The whole procedure of being alone on the island and having the whole town looking for them is filled with a great amount of libidinal satisfaction. By means of the fantasy of death the lost love relationship is restored again: afterwards everything will be all right. The same mechanism is at the basis of the usual suicidal fantasies of children and also, as we have seen, at the basis of the fantasy of this patient. By means of his death everything will come all right again—of course, he will be alive to enjoy it afterwards. Actual suicide in children before puberty is extremely rare. Probably one of the most important reasons for this is not that children do not make attempts at suicide, but that these attempts are such that they do not lead to death, because children are unable to obtain adequate means for it and also because they are looked after and prevented from doing dangerous things. The attempts at suicide made by children usually appear to be in play.

The patient whose attempts at suicide I have described acts out the suicide of a child. As he is grown up, he has adequate means at hand for committing suicide. As his sense of reality is disturbed on account of the fact that he still has an infantile belief that whatever happens his mother will save him, the precautions which he takes are inadequate. His fixation to his strong oral desires, which lead him to this particular mode of suicide, also work in the direction of making the attempts more dangerous.

In summarizing, let me state that, in this particular case, the answer to the problem I raised at the beginning is the following: the "longing to die" does not express the patient's wish to destroy himself, but serves as the expression of a libidinal fantasy. As mentioned above, the occurrence of such libidinal fantasies has been described by various writers, such as Jones (14, 15), Garma (12), Chadwick (4), M. Schmideberg (21), Bischler (2), Sterba (23). No attempt has so far been made to confront the recognized conception of suicide as the acting out of a libidinal fantasy with the recognized conception of suicide as a depressive mechanism. The mechanism of suicide in melancholia is such that the patient wants to destroy himself because the object with which he is at war is introjected and represented by his own super-ego. Therefore only self-destruction can serve the aim of the melancholiac. In the case which I have described, and also in children who have suicidal fantasies, the conflict lies not with the super-ego but with objects in the outside world. Therefore the aim is not self-destruction, but libidinal gratification by those objects by way of an attempt at suicide. Self-destruction may be the result in the child because it is not yet able to judge reality and in the adult on account of a severe disturbance of his sense of reality.

In my opinion the mechanism I have described is a mechanism not only in one particular case but one which lies at the basis of quite a number of others. The importance of an attempt to classify the various mechanisms of suicide which we meet in our patients is perhaps not so much of theoretical as of clinical interest, since the attitude of the analyst to an attempt at suicide by a patient has to vary according to the mechanism which is at the basis of the given case.

REFERENCES

1. BERNFELD, S. (1929). "Selbstmord," Z. psychoanal. Päd., 3, 355.
2. BISCHLER, W. (1936). "Selbstmord und Opfertod," Imago 22, 177.
3. CHADWICK, M. (1929). "Notes upon Fear of Death," Int. J. Pscho-Anal. 10, 321.
4. CHADWICK, M. (1929). "Uber Selbstmordphantasien," Z. psychoanal. Päd., 3, 409.
5. FEDERN, P. (1929). "Die Diskussion über Selbstmord, insbesondere Schüler-Selbstmord," im Wiener Psychoanalytischen Verein im Jahre 1910, Z. psychoanal. Päd., 3, 333.
6. FEDERN, P. (1929). "Selbtsmordprophylaxe in der Analyse," Z. psychoanal. Päd., 3, 379.
7. FREUD, S. (1917). "Mourning and Melancholia," Coll. Papers, 4, 152.
8. FREUD, S. (1915). "Thoughts for the Times on War and Death," Coll. Papers, 4, 288.
9. FREUD, S. (1910). "Schlusswort der Selbstmord-Diskussion," Ges. Schr., 3, 323.
10. FREUD, S. (1923). The Ego and the Id.
11. FRIEDJUNG, J. K. (1929). "Zur Kenntnis kindlicher Selbstmordimpulse," Z. psychoanal. Päd., 3, 426.
12. GARMA, A. (1937). "Psychologie des Selbstmordes," Imago, 23, 63.
13. GLOVER, J. (1922). "Notes on the Psychopathology of Suicide" (Author's Abstract) , Int. J. Psycho-Anal., 3, 507.
14. JONES, E. (1911). "On 'Dying Together,' " Essays in Applied Psycho-Anal., 99.
15. JONES, E. (1912). "An Unusual Case of 'Dying Together,'" Essays in Applied Psycho-Anal., 106.
16. KALISCHER, H. (1929). "Leben und Selbstmord eines Zwangsdiebes," Z. psychoanal. Päd., 3, 363.
17. KLEIN, M. (1935). "A Contribution to the Psychogenesis of Manic-Depressive States," Int. J. Psycho-Anal., 16, 145.
18. KLEIN, M. (1932). The Psycho-Analysis of Children.
19. PELLER-ROUBICZEK, L. E. (1936). "Zur Kenntnis der Selbstmordhandlung," Imago, 22, 81.
20. SADGER, I. (1929). "Ein Beitrag zum Problem des Selbstmords," Z. psychoanal. Päd., 3, 423.
21. SCHMIDEBERG, M. (1936). "A Note on Suicide," Int. J. Psycho-Anal., 17, 1.
22. SCHNEIDER, E. (1929). "Die Todes- und Selbstmordphantasien Tom Sawyers," Z. psychoanal. Päd., 3, 389.
23. STERBA, E. (1929). "Der Schülerselbstmord in André Gide's Roman 'Die Falschmünzer'," Z. psychoanal. Päd., 3, 400.
24. ZILBOORG, G. (1935). "Zum Selbstmordproblem," Int. Z. Psychoanal., 21, 100.
25. VARIOUS AUTHORS (1910). Uber den Selbstmord insbesondere den Schüler-Selbstmord (Diskussionen des Wiener psychoanal. Vereins, Heft 1).

IV. ON "DYING TOGETHER"

WITH SPECIAL REFERENCE
TO HEINRICH VON KLEIST'S SUICIDE

ERNEST JONES

In a recent interesting monograph on Heinrich von Kleist, Sadger[1] has called attention to a number of considerations bearing on the psychology of the impulse to die together with a loved one, to share death in common. As it is possible in a special journal to pursue an analysis more freely than in writings intended for a lay audience, I wish to comment here on two points in this connection which Sadger—I assume, with intention—left untouched.

Of the general psychosexual significance of the idea of death nothing need be added here. Freud, Stekel, and others have fully described the masochistic fantasies in which the idea may become involved, and this is also clearly illustrated in Sadger's monograph. The common mythological and folk-loristic conception of death as a spirit that violently attacks one mainly originates in this source.

The question of "dying together" is, however, more complicated, the tendency being determined by several motives. The most obvious of these is that underlying a belief in a world beyond, a region where all hopes that are denied in this life will come true. The wish-fulfilment comprised in this life will come true. The wish-fulfilment comprised in this belief subserves, of course, a similar function to that operative in the neuroses and psychoses; the consolation it yields, as is well-recognized by theologians, is naturally greater at times when life is filled with disappointment and sorrow. The same is true of the desire to die together with one's beloved, as is well illustrated by the accessory factors that helped to drive von Kleist to suicide.[2] With him, however, as Sadger clearly shows,[3] there was a specific and irresistible attraction toward the act, one which is not at all accounted for by the attendant circumstances. Most psychoanalysts will probably agree with Sadger's conclusions[4] that "the wish to die together is the same as the wish to sleep and lie together (originally, of course, with the mother)," and that "the grave so longed for by Kleist is simply an equivalent of the mother's bed." Von Kleist's own words plainly confirm this: he writes, "I must confess to you that her grave is dearer to me than the beds of all the empresses[5] of the world." The idea that death consists in a return to the heaven whence we were born, i.e., to the mother's womb, is familiar to us in religious and other spheres of thought.

Deeper motives connect the subject with that of necrophilia. First of these may be mentioned the sadistic impulse, which can be inflamed at the thought of communion with a dead person— partly through the helpless resistlessness of the latter, and partly through the idea that a dead mistress can never be wearied by excessive caresses, can endure without limit, is for ever loyal. The latter thought of the insatiability of the dead often recurs in the literature on vampirism; it is indicated in the verses where Heine, in his dedication to "Der Doktor Faust," makes the returned Helena say:

> Du hast mich beschworen aus dem Grab
> Durch deinen Zauberwillen,
> Belebtest mich mit Wollustglut—
> Jetzt kannst du die Glut nicht stillen.
>
> Press deinen Mund an meinen Mund;
> Der Menschen Odem ist göttlich!
> Ich trinke deine Seele aus,
> Die Toten sind unersättlich.
>
> [Thou hast called me from my grave
> By thy bewitching will;
> Made me alive, feel passionate love,
> A passion thou canst never still.
>
> Press thy mouth close to my cold mouth;
> Man's breath is god-like created.
> I drink thy essence, I drink thy soul,
> The dead can never be sated.]

In my psychoanalytical experience of neurotics, necrophilic tendencies have further[6] invariably been associated with both coprophilic and birth fantasies. Freud[7] first pointed out the connection between the two fantasies just named, and this has since been amply confirmed by most observers. On the one hand, fecal material is dead matter that was once part of a living body, but is now decomposing, facts that make it easy for an association to be formed between it and a corpse; and on the other hand it is, according to a common "infantile theory," the material out of which children are made, and, in the form of manure, is a general fertilizing principle. Love for, or undue horror at, a dead body may thus betoken a reversion to the infantile interest and fondness for faecal excrement. This explains the frequency with which the twin motives of (1) a dead woman giving birth to a child, and (2) a living woman being impregnated by a dead husband, occur in folklore, literature, mythology, and popular belief.[8] Interesting indications of both, which need not be detailed here, are to be found in von Kleist's short story, "Die Marquise von O." The same combination of coprophilic and birth fantasy probably underlay his remarkable proposal to Wilhelmine von Zenge that they should leave everything else and adopt a peasant's life; as is well known, when she refused to fulfill this "love condition" he heartlessly broke off their engagement. Sadger quotes the following passage of his in this connection: "With the Persian magi there was a religious law to the effect that a man could do nothing more pleasing to the gods than *to till a field, to plant a tree, and to beget a child.*[9] I call that wisdom, and no truth has penetrated yet so deeply into my soul as this has. That is what I *ought* to do, I am *absolutely sure.* Oh, Wilhelmine, what unspeakable joy there must be in the knowledge that one is fulfilling one's destiny *entirely* in accord with the will of Nature." I thus fully agree with Sadger[10] when he maintains that this has a hidden sexual meaning. I have further observed, though I do not know if it is a general rule, that patients having this complex often display an attitude of wonderful tenderness toward the object of their love, just like that of a fond mother for her babe; this was very pronounced in von Kleist's final outburst of "dithyrambic rapture" toward Henriette, with its "exchange of pet names that bordered on lunacy."[11]

Sadger further comments on the "traveling" significance of dying together. The connection between the ideas of death and travel is primeval; one thinks at once of the Grecian and Teutonic

myths of the procession of dead souls, and of Hamlet's "undiscov-
ered country, from whose bourn no traveller returns." The fact,
now becoming generally recognized since Freud first called attention to its importance (*Die Traumdeutung*, 1900), that children
essentially conceive of death as a "going away," as a journey, evi-
dently renders this association a natural and stable one. With von
Kleist it can be brought into line with his curious mania for traveling, which seemed so objectless and inexplicable to his friends.
Two motives in this connection lie fairly near the surface. In the
first place, death is conceived of as a voyage of discovery, as a journey to a land where hidden things will be revealed; I have had several religious patients whose curiosity, sexual and otherwise, had
been largely transferred on to this idea.[12] Sadger points out how
passionate was von Kleist's desire to reach *absolute, certain truth*,[13]
and quotes his statement: "*Education* seemed to me the only goal
worthy of endeavor, *truth*[14] the only wealth worthy of possession."
When he studied Kant's destructive criticism of the concept of the
Absolute, and of a life hereafter, he was shaken to the depths of his
being. He wrote: "And my only thought, which my soul in this
utmost tumult labored on with burning dread, was always this:
thy *sole* aim, thy loftiest goal, has declined." In the second place,
a journey can be undertaken in company, and it is significant that
in von Kleist's fugue-like escapes this was practically always so.
Sadger traces this tendency ultimately to the infantile desire to defy
the father and escape with the mother to some distant place where
he cannot disturb their mutual relations; therefore dying together
can signify in the unconscious to fly with the mother and thus
gratify secret desires.[15] The traveling mania is one of many tendencies that may come to expression in flying dreams,[16] and in this
connection I should like to throw out a few suggestions. Freud
traces the ultimate source of these dreams to the pleasurably ex-
citing chasing of childhood,[17] and has also laid special stress on
the relation between bodily movements in general and sexuality.[18]
In several psychoanalyses I have found associated with this various
anal-erotic motives, which may therefore furnish something toward the later desires. The fact itself that the common expression
for defecation is "movement," and for feces "motion," points to
an inner connection between two subjects that at first sight appear
to be quite unrelated.[19] I need not here go into the different

grounds for the association, but will only remark that when the act of defecation is especially pleasurable it is apt to acquire the significance of a sexual "projecting,"[20] just as of urine and semen. I have collected much evidence, from both actual psychoanalyses and from folklore, which I hope to detail elsewhere,[21] indicating that (a) this connotation of sexual projecting, and of movement in general, is especially closely associated in the unconscious with the act of passing flatus,[22] and (b) that this latter act, on account of the idea of penetration to a distance, is sometimes conceived of by children as constituting the essential part of coitus, which thus consists of expelling flatus into the female cloaca. The latter fantasy would, through its association with movement (and therefore flying through a gaseous medium—the air), be particularly well adapted to find expression, together with the other coprophilic, sadistic, and incestuous tendencies referred to above, in the love-condition of dying together, and I would suggest that it might be worthwhile to investigate future cases of the kind from this point of view.

AN UNUSUAL CASE OF "DYING TOGETHER"

The following dramatic event, which took place here[23] this week, seems to lend itself to some considerations of psychoanalytical interest.

A man and wife, aged thirty-two and twenty-eight respectively, went from Toronto to spend a weekend at Niagara Falls. In company with several other people, they ventured onto the great bridge of ice that forms every winter just at the foot of the Falls, and which then joins the American and Canadian shores of the river. The ice-bridge began to crack and drift from its moorings, and a river-man, who knew the locality well and who was on the ice at the time, shouted to the others to make for the Canadian side, where there was more chance of getting ashore. The couple in question ignored this advice and rushed toward the American shore, but were soon stopped by open water. They then ran in the other direction (about 150 yards), but when about 50 yards from safety the woman fell down exhausted, crying, "I can't go on! Let us die here!" The husband, aided by another man, dragged her onward until they reached the edge. This was 3 yards from the shore, and the intervening water was covered with soft ice. The river-man begged them to cross this, pointing out that the ice would prevent their sinking, and guaranteed to bring them to safety; he demonstrated the possibility of the feat by crossing himself, and later by returning to save another man. The woman, however, declined to take the risk, and her husband refused to go without her. The mass of ice now began to drift down the river, breaking into smaller pieces as it went, and slowly but surely approaching the terrible rapids that lead to the Niagara Whirlpool. In an hour's time they had drifted to where a railway bridge crosses the ravine, over 60 yards above their heads, and were on the point of being caught up by the swift rapids. A rope, with an iron harpoon at the end, had been lowered from the bridge and this was obviously their last hope of safety. As the ice-floe, now moving rapidly, swept under the bridge, the man successfully seized the rope, but apparently the woman refused to trust to it unless it was fastened around her. At all events, the man was seen to be vainly fumbling, with fingers numbed by cold, to tie the rope around his wife's waist. Failing in this in the short time at his disposal before the floe passed onwards, he flung the rope aside, knelt down beside the woman and clasped her in his arms; they went thus to their death, which was now only a matter of seconds.

These are the main facts as published in all the newspapers. The only additional ones I could discover, from a friend of mine who happened to know the couple well, were: that they were devotedly fond of each other, that they had been married for seven years, and that they, the woman in particular, were sad at never having had any children.

The husband's conduct does not call for any special comment, being dictated by sufficiently obvious motives. To these I will only add that he was in the presence of a large audience, the banks of the ravine being lined by thousands of people who had accumulated during the fateful hour, and that it would be difficult or impossible for a man to hold up his head again if he deserted any woman in such a situation, let alone his own wife.

There is, however, more to be said about the woman's conduct, or rather lack of conduct. It is evident that she was throughout overcome by panic and fright, or even convinced of the inevitableness of the fate awaiting her. Her efforts at escape were either paralyzed or else *actively hindering,* and she did not respond even to the powerful motive of saving her husband. Now it is known to psychoanalysts, as Freud first pointed out in reference to certain dreams,[24] that emotional paralysis is not so much a traumatic effect of fright as a manifestation of inhibition resulting from a conflict between a conscious and unconscious impulse. A familiar example is that of a woman who cannot protect herself with her whole strength against being raped, part of her energy being inhibited by the opposing unconscious impulse which is on the side of the assailant. The question thus arises whether any such process can be detected in the present case. If so, then the woman's conduct would have to be viewed as expressing an unconscious desire for death, an automatic suicide. The available evidence, as just narrated, is so meager that any hypothesis of this kind must necessarily be very tentative, but when correlated with psychoanalytical experience in general the probability of its being true is, in my opinion, very considerable.

There is no reason to believe that any desire for death that might have existed could have been other than symbolic; indeed the description I obtained of the woman's state of mind on the day before the calamity makes the idea of any direct suicidal intent highly improbable. We have therefore to ask what other ideas could have been symbolized by that suicide. It is known, through analysis, not only that the ideas of sex, birth, and death are extensively associated with one another, but also that the idea of dying in the arms of the loved one—*"gemeinsames Sterben"*—symbolizes certain quite specific desires of the unconscious. Of these, which have been pointed out especially by Sadger[25] and myself, one in particular may be recalled—namely, the desire to beget a child with the loved one. The unconscious associative connections between this desire and the notion of common suicide are too rich and manifold to discuss here; besides which they are now well enough known to justify one in assuming an understanding of them in informed circles. I will therefore content myself with indicating some of the respects in which the present situation was adapted for supporting this associative connection.

The association between Niagara and death, especially suicide, is one that has been enforced by countlessly repeated experiences. It is not so generally known, however, that the association between it and birth is also very intimate. Niagara is a favorite honeymoon resort—possibly more so for Toronto people than for those of other places in the neighborhood, on account of the romantic journey thither across Lake Ontario. So much is this so that Niagara town is commonly known—in Toronto at all events—as "the Baby City," from the high percentage of conceptions that date from a visit there. The couple in question were very fond of spending their holidays there, the unconscious attraction being possibly the same as that which drew women of old to the Temple of Aesculapius and which still draws women to various healing waters. They had never been there before in wintertime, a rather strange circumstance, for it is almost as popular with Toronto people in the winter as in the summer because of the beautiful ice effects to be seen at that time. It is conceivable that they were this time drawn by the idea of winter (death, cold, etc.) which was beginning to correspond with their attitude of hopelessness about ever getting a child.

Coming next to the calamity itself, we see how similar was the conscious affect investing the two ideas which we suppose became associated; the hope of giving birth to a child was almost as small as that of escaping from the threatened doom. That this doom was one of drowning—in the horrible form of being swept under in an ice-cold whirlpool—is a circumstance of considerable significance in the light of all we know about the symbolic meaning of water in general and of drowning in particular (cf. Freud, Rank, Abraham, Stekel, etc.). If the whole story were told to one as constituting a dream, one would have no hesitation in interpreting it as a child-birth fantasy of a sterile woman, the floating *on a block of ice* in a dangerous current of water, in company with the lover, in sight of all the world and yet isolated from it, the threatening catastrophe of drowning, and the rapid movement of being passively swept to and fro (above I have insisted on the significance of movement in this connection)—all this forms a perfect picture.

Though the actual situation was not a dream but a grim reality, nevertheless the circumstances detailed above are just such as would, especially in a moment of acute emotion, strongly appeal to the latent complex in question and stimulate it to activity. It should be remembered that, in times of despair (defeat, severe illness, danger, enfeeblement, approaching death, and so on), there is a universal tendency to fly from reality by having recourse to the primitive system of thought (Freud's primary *Lustprinzip,* Jung's *phantastisches Denken*), mostly in the form of infantile wishes relating to the mother; indeed I have elsewhere[26] expressed the opinion that the idea of personal death does not exist for the unconscious, being always replaced by that of sexual communion or of birth. We may thus imagine the woman in question as reacting to her frightful situation by rapidly transforming it in the unconscious and replacing reality by the fantasy of the gratification of her deepest desire. The external outcome of this act of transformation illustrates very well the contrast between the practical value of the pleasure principle and that of the reality principle.[27]

One might speculate whether the outcome would have been different if the woman's thoughts concerning childbirth had been more accustomed to assume the common form of the fantasy of saving, or of being saved.[28] It is even possible that this fantasy was operative, and that her objection to being saved by the river-man and by the men who were holding the rope from the bridge was due fundamentally to her excessive marital fidelity, to her determination that no one should save her except her husband. But at this point our speculations become so filmy as to float away into the region of the completely unknown.

NOTES

1. Sadger, *Heinrich von Kleist. Eine pathographisch-psychologishche Studie,* 1910.
2. *Ibid., pp.* 60, 61.
3. *Ibid.,* pp. 56–58.
4. *Ibid.,* p. 60.
5. Empress, Like Queen, is a well-known unconscious symbol of the mother.
6. The connection here implied between sadism and coprophilia is discussed at length in a later paper republished as chapter XXXI of the author's *Papers on Psycho-Analysis,* 2nd edition.
7. Freud, *Sammlung kleiner Schriften,* Zweite Folge, p. 168.
8. Numerous examples of this are quoted by Hanusch, *Zeitschrift für deutsche Mythologie,* Jahrgang IV, p. 200; Hock, *Die Vampyrsagen und ihre Verwertung in der deutschen Literatur* (1900), pp. 24, 37, 43; Horst, *Zauber-Bibliothek* (1821), Erster Teil, p. 277; Krauss, *Slavische Volksforschungen* (1908), p. 130; Sepp. *Occident und Orient* (1903), p. 268.
9. The italics are mine (in this instance only).
10. Sadger, *op. cit.,* p. 62.
11. *Ibid.,* p. 59.
12. One of my patients eagerly looked forward to discovering in the next world the authorship of the Letters of Junius!
13. Sadger, *op. cit.,* p. 62.
14. On the intimate association between the ideas of truth and nudity, see Furtmüller, *Zeitschrift für Psychoanalyse* (1913), Bd. I, p. 273.
15. Sadger, *op. cit.,* p. 60.
16. It is perhaps not without interest that the name of the woman with whom von Kleist departed on his endless journey was Vogel (i.e., "Bird").
17. Freud, *Die Traumdeutung,* 2e Aufl., p. 195.
18. *Ibid.,* pp. 53, 54. See also Sadger, "Haut-, Schleimhaut- und Muskelerotik," *Jahrbuch der Psychoanalyse,* Bd. III, p. 525.
19. This association plays a prominent part in the common symptom known as *Reisefieber,* and in the allied "packing" dreams.
20. It is noteworthy that the common vulgarism for the act is eymologically cognate with the word "to shoot."
21. Since the present paper was written this has been done in two monographs published in the *Jahrbuch der Psychoanalyse.*
22. It is noteworthy that the common vulgarism for this both in English and in German singularly resembles the German for travel, *Fahrt.*
23. I.e., Toronto.
24. Freud, *Die Traumdeutung* (1900), p. 228.
25. Sadger, *Heinrich von Kleist* (1910), pp. 59–62.
26. *Journal of Abnormal Psychology,* April 1912.

27. See Freud, "Die zwei Prinzipien des psychischen Geschehens," *Jahrbuch der Psychoanalyse*, Bd. III, p. 1.

28. See chapter x of my *Papers on Psycho-Analysis*, 1918.

V. THE PSYCHOLOGY OF DYING

DANIEL CAPPON

Any man's death diminishes me, because I am involved in mankind;
And therefore never send to know for whom the bell tolls; it tolls
for thee. —JOHN DONNE, *Devotions*

John Donne's lines express the general reason for writing this
article. Men of medicine have eschewed public utterances on the
dying patient. The surgeon is superstitious. He needs to be optimistic and shut out twinges of professional guilt and worry. He
turns away. The physician feels impotent. Though sympathetic,
he turns away. The psychiatrist faces often the threat of man
turned against himself; but if suicide is carried through, the psychiatrist also looks away, covered in guilt and shame. Even the
priest absorbs his keenest feelings in rituals. The relatives and
friends are immersed and blinded by grief; the nurses busy; only
the poet and the philosopher take a look from afar.

Talcott Parsons wrote, "Death, particularly premature death
is one of the most important situations in all societies, demanding
complex emotional adjustments on the part of the dying person
. . . and on the part of the survivors. This is so important that in
no society is there an absence of both cultural and social structur-
ing of ideas about death."[1] Eissler said the moments of death are
the most important in a man's life.[2]

Our cultural creed is optimism at all costs—its slogans, "Life is
for the living," and "Business as usual." We embalm the dead with
neo-Egyptian reverence, at exorbitant costs, to pay the price for
forgetting. We shift insupportable sorrow and fear, to financial
sacrifice and subsequent adulation of the marble mausoleum.
Though in bygone days, both pagan and Christian, life was transitory and death rewarding—a state worth contemplating—the atti-

61

tude of nowadays is not less understandable nor unnatural, for "Men fear death as children fear to go in the dark and as the natural fear in children is increased with tales, so is the other."[3]

Despite our cultural defenses, or perhaps because of the obliqueness with which we meet this inescapable situation, death remains unapproachable, perplexing, frightening. Only religious faith bridges the Styx, whose source lies in the enigma of mind turned to mere matter and in our wrought-up emotions regarding this great unknown. Thus it is that, as the living avert their eyes, the dying remain little understood, nor helped beyond nursing comforts.

The particular reason for this report is to examine some of "Death's ten thousand several doors"[4] so as to help, at least with wisdom, those making their exit. So they can say, "La mort ne supprend point, nous (les sages) sommes toujours prêt de partir."[5] The particular application of this study would be in the field of communication to and from the dying. When, how, what ought one to say to them, especially about their fatal illnesses? To what should one bend an ear; to what need one pay attention?

The Findings

A rather careful study was made of some twenty patients dying at a general hospital. It included a medical, social, and psychiatric assessment of their state of being. In order to draw any inferences, this group of patients was compared (qualitatively and statistically) with others who suffered not a fatal illness, and with others still who sought death by suicide. There were several startling findings:

Psychologically, the dying differed little from other patients physically ill, or, for that matter, from some patients emotionally ill with respect to their fear of death, motivation, and personality. They died as they lived; their thoughts, feelings and actions frozen by the buffetings of life in the same too often distorted, ugly patterns. Indeed, after looking objectively at what might have changed, with the approach of death, and how this might have occurred, it seemed like expecting too much. Death was conceived as a state of not-being; a change; a plunge into the unknown; therefore to most a threat, to some a release. The reaction in those seeing it as a threat was not miraculously different from all the other reactions to threats incurred before. The hostile became more hostile, the fearful more fearful, the weak weaker. They each hung on to their habitual defenses—regressing, denying, withdrawing, projecting, as before. The ego, guardian of smooth functioning, was undermined by the sapping of somatic strength, especially where death was slow to come. Consequently it weakened, contracted, or swelled to enormity, or dissolved. It did not seem to rise to the challenge of death bringing meaning to life nor to the hope of life hereafter.

Curiously, but in keeping with this challenge going on unheeded, no person dying wanted to live, at least in his present physical state. Only a few, those considered "normal" psychiatrically, wished not to die. In the rest, the deep-seated, unconscious motivation favored death—sometimes as violently as it did in others, intact in body, who wanted to bring their lives to an end. This, then, exploded the myth that everyone faced with death wants to live at all costs. In the largest group were those who went through life with a muddled mind, fearful and lonely; they found themselves on the brink of death, with nothing much to have lived for and still less to live for. Yet to themselves they denied the reality of death. They did not want to hear about it from others. But deep down, with the usual wisdom that is attributed to the unconscious, they did not want to live either. This was not as strange as it sounded for they had lived beside life rather than in it, and they were making their exit beside death, as it were, rather than with it. They did not want to die, any more than they had really wanted to live or did live; they did not want to face anything final and inevitable. But deep down they were not averse to passing on.

The psychiatrist's great difficulty in diagnosing the "normal" or even in establishing the "normative" clinically, was increased manifold when considering the dying. This was a state, abnormal at least by clinical definition, with a sure ending of which there was no clinical psychiatric appreciation. Those judged "normal" were certainly not normative, for they constituted the smallest minority group. They were relatively cheerful, their ego stronger, their communication good, and their leading psychological defense was reasoning or rationalization, for in this situation the difference between these processes became unclear. Yet, we might ask, was it appropriate to be in good cheer while dying, and could one reason or rationalize "healthily" about one's own death? The only thing one could say was that, by comparison with the "control" groups, the "normals" were more like most people considered psychologically normal under different circumstances. This is not to infer that they were exhilarated, their ego swelling, their defenses grandiose and overcompensating. There were a number like this, who were considered abnormal in that, as in other circumstances of life, they attempted to overcome prideful and pretentious obstacles.

In view of the interest of this research in communication and also in view of the fact that one had the advantage of studying the unconscious motivation of this group, the question of forebodings came up as follows: Without recourse to extrasensory perception, it was possible for all these patients dying from fatal illness, to have clear forewarnings of this fact. There were at least two avenues: One was the possibility of inner perception of an illness marching the body to the grave, increasing and combined with the many warnings issuing from outside, if not a direct opinion given by medical authority of the approaching event. The other possibility was the translation into foreboding of a deep-seated motivation or intention to die. The question was, with these two possibilities in mind, were forebodings allowed into consciousness? If so, were they more frequently allowed in those more "normal" with a stronger ego and better communication, or were they more frequently allowed by those wishing to die? This question, of course, could not be answered in a clean, straightforward way with the evidence available. The main reason was that we were not ascertaining directly forebodings but only recollected and verbally reported forebodings. Yet one might have expected some regularity even in the dynamics of this more complicated process. But this was not found. A surprisingly high number of subjects confessed having had forebodings of death. Of those who communicated at all at this level only one-third denied them. Of the ones who told of their prescience, in some it clearly coincided with their desire to die, and in this way they were indistinguishable from suicides; in others it conflicted with their alleged fear of death and desire not to die (yet not to live as they were). One of the two "normals" had formalized her forebodings into an intellectual certainty, and an acceptance that she was going to die. In the other, forebodings were denied, as they had been by those weaker in ego, fearful, hostile, or generally ostrich-like about death, as about life. Often, the denial of forebodings was so vehement that one had the intuitive empathic feeling that they were being combated with the last ounce of conscious vigor. Though there was a tendency for forebodings, acknowledged by those who communicated best, this was not always so. From some, in whom communication was diminishing to silence, these warnings would be flashed out perhaps in an attempt to have them denied by medical authority or by some other kind of authority.

After all, this was of necessity an attempt to study with still photographs a moving picture, so that one would have expected some people about to move from one mental position to another to show the unexpected response of the category from which they were just leaving or into which they were just about to enter.

When it came to assessing total communication, that is, the subject's acceptance of important communications and also his willingness to give these out, on a diminishing scale, from active, passive, partial to ambivalent or nonexistent communication, there was a remarkable correlation between ability and willingness to communicate at all levels, and good defenses against the fear of death yet acceptance of its inevitability. This was also related, in part, to the stage of dying. The pivot of this study, from the point of view of communication, was the use of sleep dream as an index of the subject's capacity to tell himself and then tell others how he interpreted what was happening both inside and outside himself. A comparison of groups of subjects ranging from those with minor somatic or psychic illness, to those with major illness of either kind, and then to those dying either from physical illness or from mental illness by suicide, showed convincingly that the process of dying was one of progressively shutting the doors of perception. Thus mental death mercifully preceded physical death whenever the process was gradual enough. This happened in both kinds of death, by suicide and by illness.

Turning now to another specific index of communication which measured the total capacity, I looked to one of importance to both "priest and doctor whom we alike adore, when on the brink of danger, not before, the danger past priest's unrequited and the doctor forgotten" (anonymous).

This was a correlation between, on the one hand, acceptance of a fatal diagnosis given to the patient and his acceptance of religion and, on the other hand, his willingness to give out on a range of progressive privacy, medical, social, and psychiatric history, then his sleep dreams, and finally, of himself to his religion. The sample chanced to be entirely Christian. In its denominational distribution it reflected the proportion in the local population, being three-quarters Protestant (the largest groups being Anglican or Episcopalian and United Church) and one-quarter Roman or Greek Catholic and Greek Orthodox.

The correlation was strikingly close: The more religion was accepted and the more the patient participated in its ministration, the more he accepted his physical fate and gave out progressively private information about himself. But the comforts of religion were not actively sought out as much as they were refused. Even in the so-called normals they were merely passively accepted. This is not necessarily a reflection of the pragmatic value of religion in the living, as it is a reflection of the avoidance of the religious, alongside similar implications of death, in the dying. Actually there was far more active seeking, without necessarily accepting, for medical information, albeit ominous, than there was for religion. But when religion was sought, the fatal verdict given by medicine was even more actively sought and accepted. In general these two receiving parts of communication, the medical and the religious, varied together. There seemed to be little difference in what Protestant or Catholic denominational category the subject was placed. Also, in general, there was far less giving out of communication than reception; and still less was given out if the information was not immediately pertinent to physical status. Finally, the less the dying gave out, the less they wanted to or could take in and the less they used what they were given.

In summary, these findings can be pragmatically applied thus: There is no rule but the rule of thumb about what to say and what to do (psychologically) with those dying; and about what to lend an ear to and to what pay attention. Yet this variability has limits and some of them we have defined here.

In the process of dying, communication is being shut off progressively, from the mental to the physical aspect of the man-entity and from "remote and deep" fantasies, to the near and shallow fantasies of body concern. A man will receive and make good use of information, say regarding his fatal illness, to the extent to which he gives out information on this and other topics. He will seek it if he really wants to know, though sometimes he will seek it when he really does not want to know. It is necessary to have an appreciation, a total estimate, of a number of psychologic factors in an individual before one can say with assurance how much he ought to be told, how much he really wants to know, and how much he can make use of. Generally this is left to the intuitive judgment of doctors, often junior doctors, and poorly informed relatives; and generally mistakes, sometimes grave errors, are made both by saying too much and saying too little. It is easier to err on the side of what to bend an ear and pay attention to—for the general rule is, "as much as time will permit." Because nowadays we are all jealous of giving time, and forget that those asking are sometimes the dying, one needs to be selective. The ear then, needs to be attuned to the sort of inner information that the patient needs to and wants to yield: his motivation in dying, his fantasies reflecting his unresolved problems, his conflicting painful emotions. At all times the ego system of defense must be taken into account and only be strained to the limit of present capacity. Generally those in attendance are afraid that the ego is weaker than it really is; or incapable of being strained by the truth. When the ego is dissolving, however, the evidence is so palpable that fewer mistakes are made.

Summary

The fear of death, allegedly the heritage of mankind despite the "colossal Christian paradox" denying it, was manifest. It was qualitatively indistinguishable from thanatophobia, because death is not represented in the unconscious; it can only be conceived as a fantasy. Man cannot soberly grasp the real, if mysterious, change to inert matter. His diffuse fear is clothed in more or less systematized myth, ideas of an after-life or nothingness. There is no experiential basis for understanding death. The only specific fear encountered once but suspected more often was that of being buried alive.

In view of the hoary omnipresence of a manifest fear of death in mankind, a survey was made by the author (and R. Banks) in the fall of 1959 in Toronto of the possible relationships between the state of fear of death, in physically intact but fearful people, and on the state of their faith. The question to be tentatively answered was: Is a manifest or latent and implied fear of death helped or even eliminated in people who profess a belief in God and/or in after-life and/or in resurrection of the body? The statements of a sufficiently large number of people were given face value and then submitted to statistical analysis. The sample contained a repre-- sentative number of Christians and non-Christians; of Protestants in adequate proportion of denominational representation and of Roman Catholics. The sample also contained a varied mixture of believers and nonbelievers. The relationship between a belief in God and a belief in after-life was very significant, in that no more than one person believing in one did *not* believe in the other. The only other definite relationship was that between being a Roman Catholic and having a more latent, repressed, symbolic rather than manifest fear of death. For the rest it seemed that there was no significant relationship: perhaps slightly more Roman Catholics professed belief in the resurrection of the body (and most Episcopalians and Anglicans did not even realize that the creed required them to share this belief); slightly more females than males believed in after-life; curiously enough slightly more of the very young or very old believed in after-life than those of mature or middle age. Regarding fear of death, there was a slight trend for those who believed in after-life to make fewer statements of fear of death than those who held no such belief, and for older people to show more overt fear of death than the younger groups. However, the strict statistical facts seemed to indicate that state- ments regarding fear of death were independent of statements of faith in God, in after-life, or in resurrection of the body. Statements of fear of death were also statistically independent of type of re- ligion or the lack of it, of age and of sex.

Turning now back to the dying, to review the largest psychological group making up the sample studied, we found they consisted of those called by Dürkheim, the sociologist of suicide, "anomic," i.e., isolated and withdrawn persons. The background of their lives revealed the bleakest possible picture. It was not unexpected that they represented the largest number, for one would think that in this age group of people dying and for this socioeconomic group found on the wards of a general hospital, the "anomic" would be the largest in number. The somewhat unexpected, however, was that a quick scrutiny of their past lives—empty, desolate, often with no other in it; no love; no pet; no values, religious or otherwise, and no interest even in a thing—and an evaluation of their present state in which what little they had in possessions inclusive of a body, was being lost; when there was nothing but the broken remnants of an animal instinct for survival to which to cling, they could not directly and consciously contemplate death. They spent their last days in blind if vague hope, unthinking as perhaps most of their days have been, and drifting into death—concerned with the immediate and therefore bodily minutiae of existence and superficial comforts. Many were in pain and, while wishing to escape it, they consciously hung on to life. As Sir Thomas Brown put it, they labored against their own cure, for death is the cure of all diseases.

The psychology of these anomic souls dying of bodily illness was in no way different from those dying at their own hands. A most dramatic finding was this correspondence between psychologic motivation in dying and the actuality of dying. Despite ego defensive maneuvers and sometimes blatant denials, many of the patients *wanted,* either passively or actively, to die. This apparent contradiction is, of course, in keeping with the usual contradictionary functionings of the mind, if one considers its different levels (conscious and unconscious), and sometimes even at the same level. One might ask then, why, if they wanted to die, trouble to hide or disguise both the wish and the actual event? The answer is that all but two concealed from themselves the two aspects of this unbearably painful state; that there was nothing to live for anyway and, worse, that death was the only solution: that they were dying and this terrifying unknown event was final and inevitable.

Contrarily to idealized belief, men die as they live—with the gall of hatred bitter in their mouths. They neither seek nor bestow forgiveness nor share in a promised peace. Their vulnerable egos, ill defended, dissolve and crumble at the sight of death. As Somerset Maugham described it in "Mrs. Craddock": "The prospect of death would be unendurable if one did not know that the enfeebled body brought a like enfeeblement of spirit, dissolving the ties of the world. When the traveller must leave the hostel with the double gate the wine he loved has lost its savour and the bread turned bitter in his mouth." Curiously, as part of the dying body, men often have a positive motivation toward death.

Though this paper makes no claim to add to thanatologies because it is dedicated to pragmatism, one can hardly escape metaphysical implication in dealing with a subject of this nature. Certainly analysis of the lives of those dying bodily, and their motivational status has analogs in those dying so many different kinds of death: the nihilism of depression, the fragmentation of schizophrenia, the psychopathic bid for the electric chair, the heroics of the Victoria Cross, the drowning in toxic drugs and alcohol, the daring of death riders on water, land or air. It is even manifest in those who destroy promising careers by their complex of "being late" for everything important. One cannot but go along with Eissler, Bergler[6] and Freud,[7] who postulate the concept of mortido. One feels that but for the mysterious *élan vitale* of Bergson, the Eros of Freud or the libido of Jung,[8] but for its last ditch cathexis in the body ego; but for the fear of yielding the psychic ego to the great unknown, the threads of life would be cut sooner rather than later by most men. The threads would be cut depending on opportunity and inclination: abandonment to potentially killing disease, abandonment to psychic annihilation or actively seeking the sundry forms of bare bodkin that might quietus make. It has been said that, from the moment of birth, life is a struggle with death. It is entirely likely that, since man is a psychosomatic construct, the death processes of catabolism should be hitched to mortido, clashing with anabolic libido, in phases, until the end when death stands triumphant. Thus the energy of life emanates from the opposition of those two great forces, personified by Eros and Thanatos. Here it may be useful to distinguish between mortido (opposed to libido) subserving natural catabolic processes, and the perversion of libido, of all life instincts, and their manifestation in positive destructive (death) drives and supported by murderous hostility which may be called "destrudo." While mortido is a theoretical construct, never manifest, always presumed in the actuality of normal existence and nonexistence, the destructive (destrudo) drives are pathological phenomena, abundantly clinically manifested. Certainly the conscious fear of death, in the dying as in the neurotic, has roots in this destructive death drive—it being an ego defense against the wish to die, blinding the self to the (Id's) person's deep wishes. This pathological perversion of life instincts, turned to destruction, is given impetus by the social structure of a person's life, by its tragic events, and given coloring by the specifics of personality. When it reaches its climax in dying and in death, there is an ultimate fusion in mortido—a fusion with all that has to perish and decay.

As for the practical matter of communication with and from the dying, the main points made in the beginning may be reiterated. These findings suggest that there is no personality change in the period of dying. Only one patient of this series made a religious and characterological conversion—stimulated by the fortuitous contact with this author, who was prying into his soul.

To determine to what one should bend an ear, and to what one should give tongue, the patient's psychiatric status, his prevalent feeling tone, his ego status, and the state and quality of ego defenses, his motivation in dying, and his forebodings, should be reviewed. Most particularly a seemingly casual attempt should be made to sample his fantasy, and his religious inclination should be observed. The gestalt obtained from this information should guide the physician, who must rely on his good sense and intuition in each individual case, when he makes meaningful contact with the patient.

In the writer's opinion, it is never justified to tell a patient a fact about his dying that the doctor perceives from an adequate study, that he truly does not want to know consciously; even to hear. Even if such neglect leads to hardship on those left behind, it is not justifiable to disturb the tenuous balance of the dying, whom one cannot help, for the sake of the living who may help themselves.

On the other hand, it is not warranted to withhold information from patients in whom adequate study reveals the need to know and to be treated as "normal" adults. One must remember that even the reality of a fatal prognosis can be a relief from the

agonizing ambivalence and struggle with the question of whether
to know whether one has to face the great unknown. Sometimes
such confirmation can bring even secret gladness and release. And
yet one must be cautious in this kind of frankness, for, as could be
seen from the study, an apparent serenity and desire to be told
does not always coincide with the real feeling. One cannot rely, as
in other instances, on the dourness or the pliability of adequate
defenses—except on the purposeful blockage in taking in communication, which, as mentioned, should never be violated.

In the last instance, one must watch the approach of the clergyman, treading lightly on the shadow of the patient's death. He will
be received according to the flickering flame of libido still integrating the ego, according to the motivation in dying and according
to the nature of defense against the final event of death. One may
mend the damage if the clergyman is waved away by the frightened
patient, or one may consolidate his strengthening ministration
with one's own brand of kindly, earthly, human ministration and
truths.

Probably the relevance of this paper does not consist so much in
its findings as in the fact that only rarely will one of us men of
medicine turn to this subject for a scientific appraisal of its varied,
frightening, and likely unfathomable implications.

NOTES

1. Parson, Talcott. *The Structure of Social Action*. New York: McGraw-Hill, 1937.
2. Eissler, K. B. *The Psychiatrist and the Dying Patient*. New York: International Universities Press, 1955.
3. Bacon, Francis. *Two Essays on Death*.
4. Webster, John. *The Duchess of Malfi*.
5. LaFontaine (paraphrased): "Death surprises us not at all, we (the wise) are
always ready to depart."
6. Bergler, E. *The Battle of the Conscience*. Washington, D.C.: Washington
Institute of Medicine, 1948.
7. Freud, S. (1920). *Beyond the Pleasure Principle*. London: Hogarth, 1948.
8. Jung, C. G. *Two Essays on Analytical Psychology. Collected Works*, Vol. VII.
London: Routledge and Kegan Paul, 1954.

VI. NOTES UPON
THE FEAR OF DEATH

MARY CHADWICK

Man fears Death as the Child fears to go in the Dark.
—FRANCIS BACON

When we come to consider the psychological manifestations of the fear of death and give careful study to the many ramifications which may be noticed in this widespread anxiety, we find that they show points in common, suggesting a fundamental origin in one of the earliest stages of human development.

One of the most remarkable phenomena of this fear is that it may frequently be found in persons for whom there is no immediate or known menace to life, when physical health is excellent, and assurances of medical opinion by no means mitigate the anxiety except for the shortest period. In consideration of this peculiarity, we may distinguish broadly *fear arising from actual danger to life, and psychological anxiety without real cause.* The former is outside the scope of this paper. Why the latter should be so prevalent and prove so devastating in its effects will be the endeavor of these notes to explain. It is interesting to notice the sublimation of this fear of death, however, in the aim of practically all medical science, to gain power over death, and to prolong life, or ease pain.

This form of anxiety, death fear, may be found among widely differing types of persons, and in both sexes. It is common at all ages, but may be rather more emphatic under certain circumstances as well as at certain times. It appears in children of a neurotic disposition far more often than is usually believed, because so many are particularly reticent upon this subject on account of its cultural connection with guilt and sin, increased by the exploitation of this fear in the training of the young by religion

73

in almost every age and among all peoples, except perhaps some of the Orientals, in whom its obverse tendency, the wish for death, may be found occupying a more important place.

Freud, in his significant work, *Hemmung, Symptom und Angst*, states that anxiety is fundamentally connected with the idea of helplessness in the infant caused by realization of the mother's absence and the fear she may never return, should she be lost to sight, which biologically includes the fear of death. He also points out the tendency to isolate the unbearable event by the interposition of a momentary blank, when anxiety is at its height, which will have the effect of making it as though it had not happened, apparently a condition of instantaneous unconsciousness, akin to that which is familiar under the name of *petit mal.* These points taken in connection with the actions and thoughts of the little child during times of stress and linked up with what may be gathered from evidence of memories of these early days in later life, from child-analysis as well as from observations of contemporary data from sick and healthy children, sometimes at a very early age, all tend to throw light upon this exceedingly complex fear of death and its complement, the wish for death.

In this way we may come to realize its fundamental alliance with the realization of helplessness, that acts as a wound to the primary narcissism of the dawning ego-structure, and we may ascertain what impressions pass through the rudimentary channels by which the infant first realizes the existence of the self and the outer world, whereby it learns to distinguish the dividing line between them. The infant must also acquire some knowledge of the conditions of life as an independent being, discover in course of time to what extent it is powerful, and how far it is helpless and where control may be exercised or when every effort against external resistance is unavailing.

Death essentially represents ʼhe power over which we have no control, a giant in whose grip we are weak, whose coming may be swift but whose summons must be obeyed. It is invisible, intangible, and therefore of a quality so unknown as to be terrifying in itself, a form of *death that is always to be feared.* The death which may be desired, however, is a self-sought death, and a condition under our own control, the act of our own will, like the achievement of Nirvana by the expert Buddhist, which is similar, except for duration, to the blank interposed by the frightened child, whose anguish eventually finds this relief.

Death anxiety, in its more superficial form, is connected with conscious guilt, by way of religious teaching and educational admonition. It is clearly a concomitant of the ego-ideal, and thus gains a conspicuous place during adolescence, when an attempt is frequently made to find relief in religious practices. We must bear in mind the close connection between adolescent guilt and fear of death which is linked by adolescent masturbation, which often breaks out anew at this time and proves a source of great anxiety to the boy or girl. The former especially will frequently receive some sort of warning, verbally or in the form of little books written for the purpose of awakening guilt, that the practice is a sin of a serious nature, causing death of the soul and often laying the foundation of physical disease which in time will also destroy the body. At a deeper level we find the boy, even without warnings from outside sources, frequently alarmed by his first nocturnal emissions at this time, as is also the adolescent girl at the appearance of blood, when the menstrual flow has not been explained to her beforehand. Both conditions appear to signify disease or impending death to the adolescent mind and awaken apprehensions accompanied with extreme guilt, which probably revive old situations of a similar type connected with masturbation or enuresis in early childhood.

From this point we may recall the importance of both these childish habits for subsequent neurotic symptoms, and their association with spoken or implied threats of castration, which brings us to another aspect of the death anxiety, that which is closely interwoven with castration fear. This fear is so closely united with death fear that it has often been described as its origin. Yet, when we come to consider the cultural sequence of the two customs in religious or penal codes, sacrificial death and mutilation, we find that the latter usually appears as a subsequent lessening of the early death penalty, which leads us to wonder whether after all castration fear may not be a derivative of the primary fear of death, which would be borne out by the equal prevalence of this anxiety in men and women, as well as its peculiar significance in each sex, which look like two branches from the same root.

Freud, in the work quoted above, *Hemmung, Symptom und*

Angst, shows these two branches clearly, when he states that the fear which proves the greatest dynamic in the life of the woman is that of *loss of love,* which acts as a full equivalent of the man's fear of the *loss of the penis.* In this case should we take the death fear as the fundamental anxiety, we may find that it may be symbolized thus:

I. *Loss of love* means separation from the parents: the child's loss of power over them, and their gain of power to bring about its destruction, death.

II. *Loss of the penis,* a second separation from the parents: also loss of the ability to return through congress with the mother in life; but the possibility of doing so in the sought death, which forms a symbolic reunion. Loss of power, no weapon with which to struggle against the armed and mighty father, which represents the dreaded and hostile death. Yet we find that in the child's mind, self-immolation wrests from the father the power to slay the son. It may also represent the loss of the self, the ego becoming identified with this organ.

Following up these steps, it seems possible to divide death into a dual representation, thus: *hostile or violent death,* the action of the cruel father, who slays the sons and orders the exposure of the daughters, unwanted father-death; and *desired, benign mother-death,* the regression to the prenatal state, wished for and neither unknown nor feared.

The woman cannot obtain the compensation of a symbolic return to the mother, as can the man, in cohabitation, even should she wish it, unless it be through identification with her unborn baby, which has been suggested by Helene Deutsch. Yet the death wish of the woman which is carried out in suicide often takes the form of a mother-regression, drowning or the gas oven. Nevertheless, we frequently find that women in whom the wish for death is the strongest, so that this expedient has been sought, have been those who have recently lost their father by death, and are so strongly fixated to him that they do not wish to continue to live without him, but in the company of the mother. In this case we see the incest-wish fantasy of union with the father in the grave (the mother), which is one of great intricacy, since it shows both hostility to the mother as well as a reunion with her, and simultaneously with the father. The mother symbol, the grave, may also serve to cancel the guilt to some extent, whereas the action itself has the practical result of escaping from the mother, who under these circumstances has probably been regarded with the keenest jealousy.

Relative to the fear of the hostile father death, it may be as well to return to the primitive customs of the world, since so many other difficulties of psychological development have been illumined by reference to aboriginal tribes. Up to the present, I believe that the effect upon the child of the primeval custom of the slaying of maturing sons by the primal father has escaped psychoanalytical investigation as one of the possible roots of fear, which still makes a prompt appearance in little children when confronted with their angry parents.[1]

The primitive father in his anger might destroy his children; among some tribes this was taken as a matter of course, in others special punishments were allotted to the murderer of his own child, which shows that it must have been prevalent but was coming into disfavor with the march of civilization, yet present-day parents may still in their anger make use of threats and punishments that show a more or less direct reference to the same idea, which call forth the cry from the child, "Then I will go away and kill myself instead." The parent who hears this will often say that he or she cannot remember the words which provoked the outcry of the child, which is an interesting example of convenient forgetting, but one may surely assume that it was something pertinent, and in the symbolic punishments still in use in the modern nursery we may find the similar idea of banishment representing death, in the sending out of the room, away from sight, into the corner, where the child cannot see others and its face is hidden, which seems regarded by the child as a serious punishment as well as by its elders. One will remember in this connection that in the Bible death is frequently referred to as hiding the face, or being no more seen, sometimes as the result of God hiding His face from those who had done wrong.

In bygone days the duration of a child's life was exceedingly precarious. The father held the prerogative to order exposure at birth among many races and could also bring about the death of sons or daughters in later years should occasion demand. Again, children could be sold, eaten or lost, which are all common themes of fairy tales, in itself a factor of no little importance. Long ago the fairy tale did not exist solely for the amusement of the children to whom it was related. It served the varied purpose of instruction and admonition as well as that of entertainment, by teaching the probable consequences of different types of behavior. The good and pleasing children were rewarded; the bad ones, those who did not please, were punished, death itself being the result in many instances of this failure, which showed the child clearly enough that to continue to please was the price to be paid for the permanence of the parents' affection and protection. Should this be lost, then life itself might be insecure.

In those early days, as shown in the fairy tales, the child would disappear in some way, be driven from home, lost in the forest, married to the first suitor who offered, whether desirable or not, like the girl in the legend married to the giant or monster, if not to death himself, while little brothers and sisters listened or looked on. Wild beasts in the mountain or a monster as in a tale might devour it, for the parental love had been forfeited. Thus love and life did very really become identified, especially in the case of the girl, whose value in the home depended upon her usefulness to her mother and her capacity to please her father.

For this reason, it is easy to see why the woman especially learns from childhood onwards that it is her duty to please, and to fear loss of life together with loss of love in connection with this capacity. We may also realize why the fear of death should manifest itself in such close union with her primary narcissism, because she knows that her beauty is a prime factor in her ability to please. It may also offer an explanation why the fear of death or not pleasing should manifest itself in such close relation with the menstrual period, which shows a diminution in beauty as well as of usefulness; and in unmarried women especially we often find it appear at this time, accompanied by a heightened craving for love. The death fear, as we have already mentioned, becomes conspicuous during adolescence (which marks the beginning of the mature sexual life), in connection with childbirth and before the approach of the menopause, which many women regard as a foreshadowing of death and fear it as such.

We may see running through all these forms of the fear of death the double thread, loss of power and gain of power, in the fear of helplessness, portrayed as a decrease of power when most needed in face of the mighty foe, or failure to please the important love-object, as we also observe in the desire for death an escape from and triumph over the enemy, which is felt to be a gain of immortal power and sometimes believed to be eternal life.

Let us now turn back to early childhood to discover there what light we may to untangle this riddle, still looked at from the dual aspects of father death, the hostile and external, involuntary and which cannot be escaped, and mother death, the desired. In the case of the girl, both may be equally hostile and expected, because of the jealousy of the mother for the daughter, on the one hand, and from the father should she fail to please, upon the other. This may indeed cause the anxiety and haunting dread of not pleasing, which is far more common in the woman than in the man; her readiness to sacrifice herself in any way if only the love of another may be retained, her frequent attitude of apology for her mere existence and her fear of incurring debt, although often trying to put others under an obligation to herself, as though in an attempt to buy back her original life-debt to her father for having allowed her to live, or to have a reserve for the future, something to fall back upon at the time of waning power and her greatest need for love, when she gets old and her beauty fades, so that it becomes not so easy to please as before.

If we take the fear of death or wish for death as the two manifestations of the realization of helplessness or desire for power on the part of the child, this also presupposes an estimation of the self in relation to an outer world which contains both benign and hostile beings, who may be controlled or placated, as well as some conception of differences whereby the outer world is distinguished from the self, in fact, a stage of ego-development sharply enough defined to resent interference and to associate this with a fear of extinction of the ego as of the person. In this case one would assume that the fear of death may be a slightly later development than the wish for death, and conversely the stage of the wish for death is a still more deep regression to the prenatal, which other writers have also shown.

From material connected with the fear of death in young children, we find that it appears in the following circumstances:

1. The result of expressions of parental anger, threats and

punishments, leading to the retort: "I'd rather kill myself!"

2. The result of death wishes against the parent, sometimes connected with squint.

3. The result of physical restraint, impeded muscular movement, calling up the cry from the child, "You're killing me!"

4. As a correlate of fear of the dark, or of becoming blind as a punishment for death wishes or masturbation.

Several of these conditions of death anxiety are familiar and have frequently been dealt with. In this paper, however, I should specially like to call attention to the third and fourth sections, *the result of physical restraint,* the value of the kinesthetic sense, which stimulates such a violent reaction and anxiety in the child, and *the connection of blindness with death,* because of the opposed and relative idea of sight and life, the eye and the ego, which appears in English children from the identical sound of the two words, eye, the organ of vision, and I, the self. Blindness as a castration symbol is, of course, only too familiar.

Those of us who have considerable experience of children and of infants know that a frequent cause of anxiety is to be unable to move, to be held fast, and not to be able to see. A baby whose bonnet, coverlet or sleeve has slipped over the eyes or hands, will often cry in unmistakable terror and struggle violently to escape.

It would seem that vision and the muscular sense, particularly the latter, are the two earliest vehicles of the dawning ego, both being rudimentary ways in which the infant may learn to control the outside world subjectively to a very great extent. Many babies discover how to exercise their omnipotence through sight. They are thus able to make objects appear and disappear at will upon many occasions, and will show disappointment when it cannot be carried out. They also experience considerable fear concerning visual hallucinations, the result of visual projection, which cannot be voluntarily controlled,[2] and they will often be led to believe that not only can they make objects disappear by the expedient of shutting their eyes, but that their eyes actually create the visions which pass before their eyes. They can turn light into darkness by this means, and are alarmed because they cannot also banish the darkness through some corresponding action of their own. This will frequently act as another cause of the fear of the dark, and may explain why Francis Bacon used this simile in his *Essay* upon death,

"Man fears Death as a child fears to go in the Dark." In connection with this fear of children connected with things seen, to exclude which they shut their eyes in the attempt to exclude or to make nonexistent, one often finds material in the associations of children and others which lead one to suppose that the mystery of the primal scene has been one over which they do not know whether to trust the evidence of their eyes. Children seem to occupy themselves with an infinity of fantasies upon this theme, the subjectivity of vision, as well as those representing the identification of the eye and the ego, and construct others relating to the tiny image of themselves which they see in the eye of another.

In passing, one may mention that a favorite excuse of parents to children who ask questions about something they have seen which they do not want to explain or acknowledge is this: "You must have been dreaming," which leads the child to doubt the evidence of its eyes rather than the veracity of the parents. The child then adopts the same form of reasoning, and plays with the idea of the subjectivity of vision at its own convenience.

Quite early do children begin to realize that death is a state of shut eyes and of immobility. The extinction of life and the cessation of vision means for them perpetual darkness, which also impedes movement. The same equation, death and darkness = closed eyes, which involves the extinction of the ego in death, seems to have been a belief that existed among the Egyptians and caused them to paint the widely open eye upon the side of the sarcophagus to ensure eternal life.

It is this idea of the extinction of the ego, which is the most intolerable factor in the conception of the fear of death. The greatest difficulty presented to the mind is to realize a negative condition, a state of nonexistence of the self or the noncontinuance of existence in relation to the outside world, which is connected to some extent with the child's early idea that things that are out of sight cease to exist, and that objects are created by their sight and exist subjectively. That the world will still continue when we are not there to see or enjoy it was one of the greatest anticipatory horrors of a patient of mine, who connected the idea of death with that of perpetual darkness and isolation, in which he could see no one, nor could he be found if lost, which was directly linked with a memory of early childhood when he woke to find that his mother had left him in his perambulator, having gone into a shop.

Fantasies of this description are to be found among those of many patients, but the following are taken from two whose development in each case was deeply affected by the death of the father in early childhood. Both believed that they were partially responsible for his death, and felt that they were to some extent also dead, for the reason that they could no longer exist in the *eyes* or *thoughts* of this parent. The father of the girl had once said, "in his eyes she was beautiful," and "she had nice eyes," therefore her beauty had ceased to exist now he was no longer there to admire her and take pleasure in it. The boy, in the other instance, identified the dead father in his coffin with his own brain inside his skull. His eyes could look down upon it, but which was the greater, the son or the father, he could never determine. Again, he felt that as the father lived on in his son, so he, being the part of his father, was now dead in him and decaying.

The child, we have remarked, may exercise some control over the environment through vision, as likewise by shutting the eyes; it may and does create the isolation or blank which serves to wipe out the undesired incidents. The baby's self-shut eyes partly control its universe, and in some cases may produce a swift regression to momentary unconsciousness, symbolic of death. The reverse of this self-blinding to shut out unwelcome sights, or again symbolically to kill an unwanted person by making him disappear, will be the contrast to the banishment punishment of the naughty child by the angry adult, together with the idea of blindness as a masturbation punishment, i.e., castration, the hostile death caused by the external force, who wishes to abolish the child from sight and life. "Get hence and be no more seen!"

Again, to return to the part played by physical restraint in the growth of the death fear. By means of the realization of pleasure through muscular movement and muscle erotism, the child learns to appreciate the power of its own ego at a very early stage of autoerotic libido development. Muscle erotism may thus take on a very high cathexis, which would lead to a correspondingly intense reaction to muscular opposition of restraint from outside sources, so giving rise to anxiety, which expresses itself as the fear of death and causes the cry, "Let go, you're killing me," in response to limitation of movement by the grip of another. This idea appears once more in the constant use of the expression "the chill grasp of death," or "in the grip of death," and recalls the action of some animals who when held tightly immediately relax every muscle, become as dead, hoping that their captor will then lose interest in an inanimate captive and throw it away.

This factor of hatred or fear of physical restraint and of interference by touch shows itself, together with the painful sensation of loss of control of the senses and muscular movement, in those who dread going under an anesthetic. In this loss of muscular control they feel that possession of themselves, the ego and super-ego is threatened. On the one hand, they will not be able to defend themselves against the attack of the operator, and they also fear "they may do something dreadful," an outbreak of the id-impulses, which would cause humiliation to the super-ego, which has been put out of control by the anesthetic. This state of affairs only too often happens in reality, as those know who have had an opportunity to observe those under anesthetics or recovering from them. Until the anesthetic takes effect, it is by no means seldom that we find the patient struggle as though for life, the shout "Let me go!" is frequent, and cases have been known when the patient has broken free and made a determined counterattack upon the anesthetist. In one of these the anesthetist, being also afflicted with a well-developed death fear, fled from the surgery and locked the door, waiting in terror outside while the patient proceeded to smash everything he could.

We may meet with this same strong reaction to the interfering touch of another in those waked from a deep sleep, or in the unconscious patient, who may be suffering from the effects of concussion meningitis, or some other acute cerebral condition. They will all show the greatest disturbance or irritability should they be touched, or the bedclothes moved so as to uncover them, a characteristic they share with persons suffering from some conditions of the graver psychoses.

In his admirable paper upon tic,[3] Ferenczi demonstrates the close connection between this muscle innervation and primary narcissism, and points out the characteristic irritability of epileptic patients and schizophrenics, who also show abnormalities of muscular movement, both spasm and deathlike rigidity, as well as stressing the relation between the psychological causes of tics and disturbances of ego-development in conflict at an extremely early level.

In reference to the correlation of primary narcissism and muscle erotism, unconsciousness as the healing blank and the phenomenon of the shut eyes as a symbol of death, I should like to conclude these notes with a few illustrations taken from a young patient of my own, a girl of fifteen, who had suffered from pseudo-epileptoid attacks since the age of seven years. She was also subject to recurrent death anxiety and showed interesting symptoms connected with shut eyes, her attitude toward father and mother, love of muscular movement in dancing, and extreme resentment of any interference with her liberty, as well as these attacks of unconsciousness, which simulated both epilepsy and death.

They would occur whenever she wished to isolate or reverse any unpleasant event, and make it as though it had not happened. She would then shut her eyes to the world and become unconscious for a time, until the anger of the relations had been changed to tender solicitude. Sometimes when unconscious she would abuse and strike the mother, accusing her of trying to kill her, and say that she would rather take her own life, since at present it was unbearable. She had also the habit of "shutting her eyes at a person," who had annoyed her past endurance, in order to banish them from sight as well as existence for her, to destroy them as definitely as she extinguished the universe and herself by her attacks of unconsciousness. The first of these, significantly enough, followed an air raid, in which she thought she was going to be killed. It was a daylight raid, and she was out shopping by herself at the time. How she ran home, dropping her parcels out of the basket as she went, she did not know, only realizing their loss when she arrived home without them. Her father was an officer in the Indian Army, to whom she was devotedly attached, a feeling he reciprocated, but she had never seen him again since she and the mother returned from India when she was about three years old. In this case, the separation from the loved father seems to have led to a profound amnesia of her whole life before this time, because she could remember at the start of the analysis nothing about her life there, nor the voyage home, except what she had been told. She had numerous fantasies of her father's return for her wedding and the presents he would bring her, one of which was to be a lace wedding veil, which recalls the interesting symbolism of ancient bridal customs.

We have here in the symptoms of this girl the wish for death, shown in the recurrent temporary withdrawal from the world, the regression to the mother, as well as the anxiety on account of her, and hostility shown toward her during the attacks, because she felt the mother kept the father away and also prevented her dancing with her boy friends, yet at the same time she feared death from the hostile soldiers as well as from some vague source, particularly at the end of each year. Each attack would be preceded by the cry: "Mother, I'm dying!" which called the mother to her side, in time for the girl to sink unconscious in her arms, but frequently during the attack she would accuse the mother of killing her and wished her to go away.

This type of regression to unconsciousness, accompanied by the expression of personal power, seen in the convulsions and epileptiform attacks of young children and infants when angry or feeling their utter helplessness, was remarked upon and likened to the quest of Nirvana by the pious, as early as 1919, in a paper read before the British Psycho-Analytical Society by Forsyth, which afterwards appeared some two years later in the *Psycho-Analytical Review,* as "Rudiments of Character-formation," and again, at the Berlin Congress in 1922, when Alexander showed the connection of the state of trance, and voluntarily developed by the Yogi with primary narcissism, in which mastery is obtained over the self, over the adverse conditions of the world and bodily pain, through a state of unconsciousness and physical immobility which is supreme muscular control, but also a condition bordering upon death and akin to catalepsy, catatonia and advanced dementia praecox.

In the early stages of dementia praecox to be found in children, it is also typical to find concurrently the fear of death, anxiety states aroused by physical restraint, muscular spasms and hypercathexis of muscle erotism, showing itself in repeated rhythmical movements, the prevention of the continuance of which will generally produce extreme irritation or anxiety. In the characteristic fantasies of these children we find, not only the themes of regression to a prenatal state of immobility, but also those of violence directed against another, generally the father, or suffered by the self from a hostile foe, that is, both *death wishes* and the *fear of death*.

It is common to find in children with whom this fear of death has reached a high development, together with the death wishes, rituals of magic by which not only shall the death of those whom they fear be accomplished, but also rites of reanimation for the reversal of the death wishes of others as well as themselves. This, in point of fact, represents the attempt to gain power over the almighty force, death, to hold in their own hands the control of death and the reanimation of those whom they have condemned to die. This being accomplished, they seek further rituals or fantasies of procreation and self-procreation, in fact, all the acts of God, to whom the power of life and death is ascribed, in which case they would be more powerful than the parents themselves.[4]

Many children will find a means of producing a temporary stasis in mind or of physical anesthesia by intense rigidity, the simulation of death akin to that of the trapped animal to escape from the hostile grip of an enemy, which the animal produces by the opposite mechanism, muscular relaxation. Muscular control of this kind gains the power that is sought, a compensation to the primary narcissism, in fantasy if in no other way, to spare them the anguish of humiliation in acknowledging a power greater than their own, which in itself will provide anxiety, and call forth this feeling of menace to the ego, which afterwards crystallizes into the fear of death, because they believe that to yield will mean death or captivity of the ego, their own loss of power or love, reinforced with primitive death wishes against this stronger foe, provoking unconscious guilt and fear from those far-off times when the father met the opposition of the child with death.

NOTES

1. See *Difficulties in Child Development*, Chapter XII, "Both Sides of the Oedipus Conflict," by Mary Chadwick (Allen & Unwin).
2. As Forsyth pointed out in his paper "The Infantile Psyche: With Special Reference to Visual Projection," published in the *British Psychological Journal*, April 1921.
3. "Psycho-Analytical Observations on Tic," *International Journal of Psycho-Analysis*, Vol. II, 1921.
4. Cf. Ernest Jones, "The God Complex," *Essays in Applied Psycho-Analysis;* also Mary Chadwick, "Gott-Phantasie bei kindern," *Imago*, XIII, 1927.

VII. PSYCHOTHERAPY FOR THE DYING

HATTIE R. ROSENTHAL

Fear of death, as a significant experience, is probably felt by most people in our Western civilization. In our youth, and as long as our expectations and hopes seem likely to be fulfilled, thoughts and fears of death are usually covered up. As Zilboorg (1) writes: "In normal times we move about actually without ever believing in our own death, as if we fully believed in our own corporeal immortality. We are intent on mastering death . . . we marshall all forces which still the voice reminding us that our end must come some day, and we are suffused with the awareness that our lives will go on forever. . . . We must maintain within us the conviction that we are stronger than all those deathly dangers, and also that we are exceptions whom death will not strike at all."

This psychologic defense mechanism, however, tends to break down when we are overwhelmed by the anticipation of catastrophic developments. Zilboorg says: "The anxiety neuroses, the various phobic states, even a considerable number of depressive suicidal states and schizophrenias demonstrate the ever-present fear of death which becomes woven into the major conflicts of the given psychopathological conditions. In these conditions the fear of death is displaced to or connected with a number of fantasies which are . . . nonrealistic."

As a rule, people seek psychotherapy because they cannot cope with the everyday problems of life. It often develops that, among other fears, they are beset by a diffuse fear of death, or unconsciously have the wish to die. A person who finds himself in a crucial conflict and does not see any way out, may unconsciously regard death as the lesser evil and use it as an escape from the problem. At first glance it might appear strange that one should have an unconscious wish to die, especially since we are used to considering the unconscious part of our personality as linked with instinctual, that is, biological drives. Here we enter the field of what Freud (2) called the Death Instinct. The therapist must respond to the patient's irrational fear of death or wish for death in a rational way, and try to alleviate or eliminate the underlying causes.

Yet there is another, small segment of people with death fears which I should like to call the "forgotten" patients — those who have been stricken by a fatal organic disease, such as multiple sclerosis, leukemia, or the great variety of cancer syndromes, and who realize that their time is running out. In such instances, we cannot speak of irrationality of the death fear. We are dealing with the patient's specific fear of the actually impending death.

When such a patient is pronounced incurable and is expected to die — within weeks or months or even years — medicine comes to his aid, ready to relieve his physical suffering. But what is done and what can be done about his mental suffering?

Taking up therapy with a dying patient, the therapist's first task is to find out whether the patient has been informed of the fatality of his sickness (some physicians prefer to inform their patients of their true condition) or whether he is semi-aware or unaware of the seriousness of his illness. The therapist will then direct the therapeutic process along the lines of this knowledge.

Family and friends can seldom give the patient the expert psychological support he needs. As a rule, those closest to him try to dispel his fears by avoiding all discussion about his illness, or if they do discuss it, they try to pretend that he will get well. The patient who, nevertheless, has his serious doubts, or can read his fate on his relative's faces, is forced to internalize his fears of death. They become tabooed subjects and, subsequently, the patient begins to fear his fears, which are intensified by the projected anxiety of his family and friends.

References in the literature to psychotherapy for the dying are few and far between. Eissler (3) writes: "the magnitude and the gravity of the situation must be fully recognized, acknowledged and accepted. . . . It is immaterial whether the patient knows consciously or not that death is impending. Somewhere within him there is such knowledge." Eissler believes that if the therapist were to behave toward a patient who has no conscious knowledge of his impending death as he would toward one suffering from a benign disease, he would probably not elicit a favorable transference reaction. "Despite the patient's alleged — and from the point of view of consciousness his true — ignorance of his condition, I believe that most patients would sense the incongruity of [the therapist's] behaviour."

Whether a patient is fully aware of his condition or not, the therapist can play an important role in this situation. Unlike family and friends, he can deal with the patient's fears rationally, with warmth and yet with detachment, and bring him tangible relief; unlike them, he enables the patient to verbalize and to face his fears. Instead of suggesting to "forget," he encourages him to "remember." For one of the therapist's primary goals is to bring hidden fears into awareness and to work toward their resolution.

In addition to the anxiety created by repressed fear, the dying patient often experiences the feeling of being rejected, shunned, and abandoned, as though he no longer belonged to the living. This observation is often fully justified, inasmuch as many relatives are so overwhelmed by the impending disaster that they are unable to cope with this situation and may prefer to withdraw entirely from the unbearable scene. The following are two examples of patients in whom feelings of being abandoned were pronounced:

A forty-seven-year-old woman suffering from cancer of the breast gave vent to her feelings three weeks before she died, by saying: "They [my family] have already given me up. They have divorced themselves from me. They are even afraid to talk to me. If at least I could say good-bye to them!"

A fifty-one-year-old man with a severe coronary thrombosis revealed his feelings in the following dream: "Many people were standing around a big hole in the midst of a patch of green meadow. All were silent. The silence was oppressive to me and I wondered why there was no talking, no hand-shaking. Finally I left in anger and determined never to see them again."

The dying patient often has an underlying strong feeling of guilt—his guilt toward his relatives which grows in intensity with every hour that brings him closer to death. Some of the religiously inclined patients see themselves confronted with the Lord's High

Tribunal before which they have to stand trial for their moral trespasses. On the other hand, the patient's relatives may see in the dying person's anxiety their own projected guilt feelings and may be greatly disturbed by a sense of having at one time or another wronged or mistreated the patient.

It appears that the patient's guilt feelings represent one of the most potent elements behind his fears of death. They should be the therapist's primary concern.

The dying patient often tries to obtain relief from his death fears through confession, which absolves him of his conscious feelings of guilt. However, relief gained from confession differs greatly from relief obtained through psychotherapy, both in nature and duration. Confession relieves his conscious guilt feelings through an act of divine forgiveness imparted to him by an external agent, the clergyman. The priest may tell him that God has forgiven his sins, the real and imagined ones. This may be sufficient for some patients whose main concern is to have made peace with their God. Yet we know that in many cases inner peace can be obtained only if guilt feelings are resolved from within—not merely by an act of forgiveness from without. A clergyman may give comfort and support. Psychotherapy, on the other hand, by dealing with the dynamic sources of guilt feelings, can bring about insight and help to resolve the guilt. Without some degree of insight, guilt feelings, although they may be repressed, are likely to remain an active and potent source of continuous anxiety.

Below are some of the specific problems that may cause the dying patient acute suffering and thus become a subject of therapeutic endeavors:

The Unfulfilled Self. Any patient whose conscious thoughts revolve around his death is inclined to contemplate on his past life, trying to account spiritually for his actions or lack of them. If he believes his life to have been a failure, to have fallen short of self-fulfillment, he may be overcome by a painful feeling of frustration. The following may serve as an illustration:

A forty-five-year-old woman was suffering from an incurable uterine cancer. She had been married for 26 years. Her husband, a lawyer ten years her senior, was a perfectionist who made her life difficult. Her twenty-three-year-old son, an obsessive-compulsive character, emulated his father in every respect. When the patient began to be aware of the seriousness of her condition, she became depressed and withdrawn. In therapy, undertaken at her husband's request, the chief objective was the patient's complaint that her life had been a total failure. She had considered her good looks as her only asset and had constantly tried to capitalize on it. Her husband, she felt, had always tried to undermine her self-esteem, which was now very low. She had at all times been so preoccupied with her appearance that she had missed many of the things that make life worth living. She blamed her parents and her husband for their failure to give her the incentives to strive for the higher values of life.

The patient experienced considerable relief after verbalizing her hostility toward her parents, her husband, and the world at large, a hostility of which she had been only partially aware prior to therapy. She realized that her life, as it was about to be terminated, had not been a failure and a waste. On the contrary, she was able to see that, although she had not always been fully aware of it, her life had been a successful one; she had actually been a good wife and mother considering the trying circumstances under which she had had to manage. Gradually she reached the point where she could look back on her life as an accomplishment and one that had been worth living. Gaining this new perspective of herself served toward a strengthening of her ego at this late stage.

What is the value of bolstering the ego when life is in the phase of final deterioration? The person with the weak ego feels that he or she has been living on the useless side of life and he regrets not having made better use of himself. This makes dying a premature process for him and he suffers from the fact that he can never make up for his lost chance. "A strong ego does not mind dying," says Gutheil (4).

The "Tragic Guilt" Feeling. In some cases, in which a patient's mother was ill or died in childbirth, he may have unconsciously carried with him a guilt feeling throughout his life. He himself may yearn for death as a just punishment for his "guilt"—an attitude (conscious or unconscious) which Flanders Dunbar (5) calls being "half in love . . . with death." Here we may describe the case of a man who was afraid that by getting married and having children he would destroy another woman's health, as he believed he had destroyed that of his mother. The uncovering of his motives removed the torturing effects of his guilt feelings:

A sixty-five-year old architect suffered from leukemia. He had always entertained the wish to die and had always been afraid of marriage. His parents were middle-aged when he was born, and he remembered his mother, who died when he was six years old, as always being sick. When he was five, his father once told him: "Your mother was never sick until you were born." In his dreams, the idea of his father blaming him for his mother's death and his taking the blame on himself was clearly expressed. He felt that he had destroyed his parents' happiness by the fact of his existence and he did not want to add to this guilt by causing the death of another woman, should he ever marry. Analysis revealed that the choice of his career, his working "constructively" (as an architect), had served to counteract his self-destructive wishes. Working through hitherto unverbalized emotions and understanding their origin and meaning greatly relieved his feeling of misery. At this late stage of his life, he was enabled to replace his crippling feelings of guilt by increased self-acceptance.

We must not overlook the fact that when insight is gained on the threshold of death, the frustrated patient will almost invariably perceive his life as not having been wasted. Eissler (3) writes: "In the presence of terminal maximum individualization a person may discover that he squandered a treasure and he may be seized by the greatest regret. But . . . this recognition may lead to a triumph of individualization, and the final processes of structurization during the terminal pathway may provide the past life with a meaning which it would never have acquired without them."

Fear of Loss of Power. One strongly pronounced component of the dying patient's fear of death may be the awareness of losing his power over his destiny. The more dominant, the more aggressive the individual was in the past, the stronger will be his fear of death. A rebel in life is a rebel in death. Just as he did not submit in life, so he does not yield in death without intensive struggle. Conversely, the man who has always been submissive and humble, or was fatalistically resigned to the demands of living, is better prepared to face death, to give up his life with less of a fight and even with less fear.

A fifty-eight-year-old man with carcinoma of the prostate was terrified by the knowledge of his coming death. Initial interviews revealed that he had for many years been the victim of a neurotic phobia—the fear of losing his potency, a phobia that was exacerbated as a result of his prostatic difficulties. He significantly identified death with a castrator. Psychotherapy helped him to correct his irrational ideas about death.

Fear of Death versus Creative Activity. One way to reduce the patient's fear of death is to rearouse his creative impulses. Many dying patients become completely passive and just wait for the end. In the case of a painter or writer, the therapist can be of immeasurable help by reactivating the patient's interest in creative activity, whether this results in purely intellectual pursuits or in actual performance. The beneficial effect was apparent in the following case:

A sixty-two-year-old painter discontinued work when his illness (hepatitis) was found to be incurable. During the last few weeks of his life, under the influence of therapy, he began to paint again and produced a striking picture which he entitled "The Destroyer." Therapy had made him see why he should not give up and convinced him that he was still creatively articulate. Moreover, the fact that he was creating something that would last beyond his death—thus annulling its effect, as it were—instilled in him a sense of immortality.

When a patient is dying, psychotherapy, like medicine, cannot achieve a cure. At best, it can provide relief and support. While the therapeutic goal differs from that applied in disease, the technique remains the same. A dying man is still an individual with needs similar to though not identical with those who go on living. To be sure, time is the essential limiting factor; the destruction of the body may have gone too far to be stopped. Psychotherapy, while unable to prolong life, has a life-sustaining and enhancing quality. It can bring about greater self-acceptance and existential reconciliation. In treating the neurotic, the therapist's goal is to convert destructive feelings into constructive, creative self-realization. In treating the dying patient, the goal is to resolve the negative feelings toward himself and his past. The therapist helps to develop in his neurotic patient the courage to come to grips with the problems of his past, so that he can face the future with changed attitudes and expectations. The dying patient has no future, but the therapist can deal with his past and try to eradicate or diminish feelings of worthlessness and futility.

We see here a seemingly paradoxical phenomenon. Viewing the situation superficially, we might be inclined to assume that the person who finds his life futile, would face death with eagerness. The opposite is true. It is the person who is convinced that he has lived a full life who is ready to die, and who develops comparatively little anxiety. A significant desire to die can be found in the psychology of melancholia, which, however, shows an entirely different psychodynamic structure and cannot be used as evidence in cases like ours. In melancholia, the patient's *élan vital* is sick: a condition of *taedium vitae* exists. Due to this, disease and death appear under all circumstances as an improvement and as a welcome solution. In the dying patient, it is not his approach to life but his approach to death that has to be reconstructed.

The technique is similar to that used in the treatment of the neurotic patient. In the initial interview a good rapport should be established and the patient made to feel free to express his thoughts. Subsequently, the therapist must try to uncover and understand the patient's past "style of life" (6) and try to afford him insight through clarification and interpretation. This "has to do not so much with the positive quality of being courageous, but rather the negative quality of not becoming discouraged" (1). Obviously such therapy must be confined to those who in their last phase of life are still amenable to insight and ready to come to a recognition of their true self, to correct their parataxic distortions, who want to achieve real inner peace. In this approach death is felt to be an integrative process, a return to and union with the universe. In general we may say that once the patient's feelings of fear, guilt, and hostility have been resolved, at least in part, he will find it less unbearable to accept the inescapability of death.

The therapist must, of course, be aware of the potential danger of insight therapy to the dying patient. He must evaluate the person's remaining ego strength and his readiness to touch upon vulnerable areas which had been repressed. He will have to weigh the advantages against the disadvantages in the light of each individual case.

Why should a dying patient have psychotherapy, when his time is so irrevocably limited? All psychotherapy is designed to help the patient cope with the contingencies of life; but in a broader sense it is also preparation for the acceptance of death. If it makes it easier for the living to live, it can also make it easier for the dying to die. For the therapist this is a great challenge.

BIBLIOGRAPHY

1. ZILBOORG, GREGORY. "Fear of Death," *Psychoanalytical Quarterly*, Vol. 12 (1943), p. 465.
2. FREUD, SIGMUND. *Beyond the Pleasure Principle*. Transl. by James Strachey. New York: Liveright, 1950.
3. EISSLER, K. R. *The Psychiatrist and the Dying Patient*. New York: International Universities Press, 1955.
4. GUTHEIL, EMIL A. *The Handbook of Dream Analysis*. Boston: Liveright, 1951.
5. DUNBAR, FLANDERS. *Mind and Body*. New York: Random House, 1947.
6. ADLER, ALFRED. *What Life Should Mean to You*. Boston: Little Brown & Co., 1931.

VIII. DEATH—
THE GIVER OF LIFE

JORDAN M. SCHER

In the course of a period of duty as Psychiatrist of the Cook County Jail, I had occasion to become quite intimate with a number of the prisoners on the so-called death row. Among these were two men who had been accused of killing policemen and a third who had been convicted of killing a factory guard in the course of a robbery. I grew to know each of these men quite intimately over the course of several years prior to their disposition from the jail. Two of the men were electrocuted and a third became the subject of a now famous Clemency Board ruling releasing him from the threat of death by electrocution. The names of the first two men were John Carpenter and James Dukes and the third was Paul Crump.

I watched Carpenter over several years while he was continually kept in solitary confinement on the ward for mentally disturbed patients. Carpenter's world seemed to have become focused down to the very narrowest. He was able to squeeze intricate details out of the extremely sparse items within his small cell. He would stand for as long as I would allow him to and describe for me that "a cup is for coffee. You put a cup into your hand and you take the cup to where the coffee is, then you pour the coffee. You take a sip, walk around, put the coffee down. You don't want to take too many sips, because it will be gone." He usually referred to himself through the use of the third person or the first ultimately, saying for example, "he got the chair." "You know he is going to get the chair." "They are going to put me in it." "They say I shot a man and they are going to give me the chair." Carpenter would stand for hours contemplating his cup or some other aspect of his environment. There was some question regarding Carpenter's competence for the purpose of execution. It seems that somehow it isn't "cricket" to execute a man who is not in his right mind since he may not experience the full force of society's judgment. Nonetheless, Carpenter was not a sympathetic figure in any sense of the word, since he was a lean, shabby loner who attempted neither to make new friends nor directly enlist anyone in his behalf.

Carpenter was found sufficiently sane for the purpose of execution and he was accordingly electrocuted. At the last moment, as Carpenter was about to leave his cell for the electric chair, he took off one of his shoes, tore the heel from it, saying "I am doing this so no one else will have to stand in my shoes." Perhaps Carpenter was sane and not psychotic. Perhaps Carpenter even had a final touch of altruism. Perhaps he wanted to reach out to those who could hear.

James Dukes was a thirty-eight-year-old Negro who had killed an off-duty policeman under bizarre circumstances. While under the influence of drugs and/or alcohol, he became involved in a tragic comedy of errors. Carrying a pistol for no clear-cut reason in his belt, while going to church to see if his girl friend was there, he was accosted and obstructed by several of the ushers who observed his state of mind. An argument trailed down the next block, caught the notice of two off-duty policemen. The policemen, in order to quell the disturbance, attempted to stop Dukes, who then fled. A series of shots was exchanged, and one of the policemen fell mortally wounded.

At the time of the execution of Dukes, there was still in the minds of some a question as to whether the bullet which terminated the life of the policeman had been fired by Duke's gun or by that of the policeman's partner since the stricken officer had been in a position between the other two. The question seems to have become settled for all practical purposes with the execution of Mr. Dukes, despite the fact that the only bullet found near the dead man was a police .38 slug—a bit of evidence which only came out in the third trial of Dukes and was discounted.

During the last few days of Dukes' life, I became a close attendant on him: one might almost say specialed him psychiatrically, to use the nurse phrase. Dukes and I talked about many things including his previous background and the history typical of a deprived southside Chicago Negro. He seemed to feel that he regretted really nothing he had done or in which he had been involved.

We talked of the fact that, in the course of his apprehension, he had been next to death as a result of a bullet wound inflicted by the surviving policeman as well as his account of police brutality later in extracting a confession from him. Dukes wondered why they worked so hard to preserve him only to finally electrocute him.

While in jail, Dukes had educated himself and had with him at the last a copy of Plato's *Dialogues,* from which he quoted a line in the *Crito* where Socrates said as he was taking the hemlock, "Do not look so concerned, my friends, they can kill me, but they cannot hurt me." Dukes was interested in the nature of life and death as we sat there in the two or three days before his execution: "What is it all about?" he asked, "What is it really for? What is man all about? Tell me, Doc, tell me, what is man all about?" I could only reply inanely, "I don't know, what do you think?" We talked about life and death. We talked of the very fine shoes another prisoner had given him. Dukes felt he was a young man in the prime of life and still had sensual desires. He wrote a letter which I include as follows:

> Man's final test in life. From the beginning of comprehension, subconsciously and unconsciously, man is constantly testing his ability to endure and adjust. His achievements and failures are usually balanced but, each one knows there is a supreme test. What would be his actions and reactions should he know the exact hour of death? Many come and go yet never know. Every day they strive to make preparations for the inevitable through various religious denominations or within their own selves. Influenced, pushed and even bribed to such an extent he is constantly wandering around in a state of perplexibility. Now I find myself facing man's final test. How do I feel? Honestly, I can't say. Scared, yes, nervous and even forgetful, wondering about the unknown.
>
> Perhaps it might be different if I felt this end was my ultimate and just good. Even if the law which we live by had been applied properly and correctly, unbiased in my behalf, I could say this is God's will, though, I must pay for my misdeeds. But this is a grave injustice, because as I sit here now I know and also the officials know there is no positive proof as to who really killed officer Blyth that night.
>
> They say two juries found me guilty and that is true. But are laymen qualified to weigh the legal technicalities of a crime of passion or premeditation? And what could their decision be when they have only heard evidence against the defendant and none for him. I

understand the State has a job to do but to what extent are they supposed to stretch the law? Where does dedication to duty end and moral obligations to humanity begin? Can they honestly and truthfully say, "I" have been fair and there is no doubt in my mind about this person being guilty of the alleged crime or have "I" used (interruption, the news broadcast just stated my last hope was denied).

It is now useless to continue talking about a people who will never divorce barbarism from their souls. Judas should be a saint in comparison to the people who are supposed to represent our society as a whole. I have approximately thirty-six hours to live. Precious, valuable time and how should I apply it. Bitterness, forgiveness, or hopelessly hoping for a lost cause. None of these seem appropriate, maybe forgiveness, because it is not for me to judge, tho I have been judged somewhat harshly.

Oh you sweet life, cruel, bitter tantalizing mistress of creation, you knew what my destiny was from the beginning of time. Is it true I am supposed to be the master of my fate and captain of my soul. Looking at it objectively, I can easily say yes but the laws of nature won't let me leave it there. Nature is "Supreme" and she alone has set up the many walks of life and the moment we try to use the so called "common sense" in preference to our "instinctive powers" we are bound to make mistakes. Since most of our convictions are influenced by convention, we are no more or less than puppets, tools and instruments used by superior minds to substantiate their aggressiveness in a field of fame and glory. So I would say basically we (the common person) live and die without ever fully realizing just what our purposes are in life. Even the few moments of happiness are surrounded and over-shadowed by a subconscious fear of what's around the next corner. I read where one philosopher said it is impossible to achieve a complete state of happiness.

Right now I'm in a state of dejection, feeling sorry for myself but where are the tears? For a minute I had my head hung in despair but this is no good. How can I expect the many good people (laymen basically) who are pulling for me and will continue to do so, to feel I gave up now.

A song is playing on the radio. "I'll Never Be Free." Will I be free even in death? Will the people who prosecuted so vigorously be satisfied after my death?

It's funny how a light weight conversation, spiritually or generally, can up lift the spirits. Even with the threat . . .

Dukes never finished his letter and in the last hour of his life, I was replaced at his side by a Catholic priest. When I left him for the last time, I caught myself saying to him at a moment when no word could possibly cover the situation, "Good luck." He returned my wish and smiled in gentle irony. Each of us felt that in this life at least, I would have a better chance for good luck than he. But then maybe not.

I had made up my mind that I would watch the execution since I had never had such an experience. I felt that to more clearly understand the meaning of death, or the theft of life, I would be a party to it. I watched the electricians busying themselves .with final tests on the chair. They seemed to fumble nervously and one of the guards commented, "'Union help, you know, Doc."

Within the last hour, witnesses and observers gathered. White benches, borrowed from the chapel, were reserved for the sheriff, official witnesses and witnessing doctors. The witnesses were supplied a folded white towel with which to wipe their brows in case of need.

I was given a front-row seat a few feet from the chair. Around me were the reporters from the various papers assigned to cover the story. All exhibited an edge of "giggly nervousness" and "gallows levity." The warden addressed the reporters saying, "You all know the rules and none of you have cameras hidden in your tie or behind your balls." This set off a round of further tittering and stepped up the general feeling of gaiety and humor alive in the air. At the warden's suggestion, watches were synchronized and a description of the duration and procedure given. Dukes was to be executed at 12:05 and would receive two jolts of 19,000 volts of electricity with an interval between them of lower voltage.

The room in which we sat was very hot and steamy from the bodies of reporters closely packed on the bleachers. A glass screen, normally in place between the chair and ourselves, was raised as the house lights dimmed at 12:02 A.M. The area of the chair was bathed in light from several spotlights placed around it. The audience now quieted and grew tense. Within another moment, two heavy officers entered half carrying Dukes from the small door to the right of the chair. His head had been hooded in black and his pants had been cut off about three inches above his knees, hastily and irregularly with a knife or a pair of scissors.

I did not realize how short Dukes actually was until I saw him stumbling and shaking toward the chair guided on either side by two guards. The entire routine had been practiced so that each guard knew his place and role and each moved quickly to complete his task. Very rapidly, Dukes was strapped into the chair, an iron clamp over thighs, upper arms, wrists and ankles, a steel band across his chest. The captain of the guards standing about three feet to Dukes' left raised his right arm and, with a gesture not unlike that used by starters in track meets, lowered it to signal the beginning of Dukes' end. At the same time, he removed his hat with his left hand and held it across his chest. If Dukes said anything at that moment, I did not hear it.

Almost immediately, his arms and legs moved into a flexor spasm and his chest pressed forward against the steel band around it. He looked like a man sitting in a chair in an awkward fashion, tensing his arms and legs, as though straining at stool. The current, as promised, was relaxed, then brought full and again he tensed. The scene was both terrible and anticlimactic since, aside from the knowledge that he was dead, he seemed to be sitting in the exact manner as he was in the beginning of the procedure. A faint wisp of blue smoke rose from where his right calf had touched the electrode and had possibly been seared.

A thin stream of blue liquid ran down his neck and chest from the copper sulfate sponge that had been placed atop his head, like an overgrown mushroom. The chief guard tore or cut his undershirt strap so that the doctors might certify an absence of pulse and respiration.

Throughout this entire procedure, the Catholic priest had stood a foot or two beyond the captain of the guards, who was very close to the chair. The priest uninterruptedly continued droning incantations and prayers. I wondered whether he saw in this death anything different from death in bed or under other circumstances. The metal and glass screen clanked down again into place.

The house lights were turned back on and the reporters busied themselves talking to the doctors, the warden, the priest and some of the guards. A press conference and some food were available in the warden's office and those with the stomach for them went. I did not, nor do I believe my role in Dukes' last days received any public notice. One reporter, very excitedly, asked me as I was leaving the building, "How did he feel, Doc, when you saw him, was he depressed?" I merely shrugged and moved off.

The third condemned man, Paul Crump, was said to have been a "model prisoner" and many agitated for a commutation of his death sentence. Crump was suave, obsequious, haughty, and highly verbal. He was said to be rehabilitated according to *Life* magazine and the general thesis of many well-wishers and do-gooders. The front office at the jail held Crump in high esteem and satisfaction. There were rumors, however, that Crump maintained order on his tier with a savage, if not sadistic hand, and that he seemed able to achieve a transfer to his tier of attractive, young homosexual men who caught his eye.

Crump's friends, feeling he was rehabilitated, convinced the parole board and the governor that he was rehabilitated. I was perhaps the only demurring witness who had seen him professionally. Had Crump been running for a political office, the entire program that saved him from electrocution could not have been better publicized and managed. Crump, of the trio, did not die. In fact, he had written a book which was published subsequent to his commutation. It is curious that Dukes, who appeared before the clemency board about two weeks after the Crump decision, with considerably less fanfare, was asked whether or not he had written a book. One wonders what might have happened if he had.

I have gone into some details concerning my participation at certain points in the lives of three human beings. With Carpenter, I was only a bystander; with Dukes, I came as a late and last friend; with Crump, a skeptical and reluctant witness.

Why have I discussed these episodes in the game of life and death? Death must be viewed in at least two ways. One is the simple event of physically dying, or ceasing to be an active participant with others in the world. The second way of viewing death is far more intriguing and subtle. I am speaking here of the mystic and, certainly, primordial, i.e., the breaking of the band of life to life. To understand the latter, one must take in, in the fullest sense, a concept of life as held in the primitive mind of all ages, the witching mind of not so long ago, and the still persistent finite-holding mind of so-called modern man. For each of these there is only a fixed, definitive—neither reducible nor expandable—quantity of life or life stuff available to those holders of it.

Since Cain slew Abel, and even before, when man slew beast, the mantle, the birthright, the very life stuff of the vanquished or the slaughtered was somehow mystically acquired in a strangely concrete way by the victor or the hunter. It was not uncommon for Greek warriors to eat the heart of a brave and fallen enemy so that they might absorb his strength. It is a not unpopular saying in today's world that if you eat fish, you will have more brain power or if spinach, you will become stronger. Witchcraft was deeply alive with the concept of acquiring, tampering with, controlling, or changing the life stuff of another. Men fear traffic with the dead (and those who conduct such traffic*). The evil eye is still feared today since men think it capable of great powers of destruction or control of the life stuff. Even the psychiatrist is feared since it is rumored he can see into and control this life stuff or psyche.

Genocide, or the destruction of one ethnic or culture group by another, is a clear-cut modern reflection of the ancient myth that the death of another means the enhancement of life for oneself, or returning of surplus life stuff to the reservoir from which it can then be reassigned. Hitler clearly was freeing up, in his strange view, life stuff from inferior repositories such as Jews, Slavs, etc., for more appropriate use by the master race.

Is there something similar between the state destruction of James Dukes and the private destruction of the three recently murdered civil-rights workers in Mississippi? Even if Dukes had put his man to death, what could it possibly avail to send him to that place also; unless one holds that those who have transgressed against conventional standards of life-holding must then forfeit a proportion of their life stuff commensurate with the degree of their transgression (an eye for an eye, a tooth for a tooth, a life for a life). What could it avail the conspirators who assassinated the three civil-rights workers or in the elimination of Dukes? Certainly there is nothing accomplished either in trials or death sentences that alters in any significant way the life of a community aside from institutional reciprocity and retaliation.

There must then be a *mythical* reason for the snuffing out of

---

*So special is our relationship to manifestations of the "All" or the Divine, i.e., the source of life substance, that it was deemed a contamination to touch directly the Torah of the Jews, since it represented the work of the hand of God, life-giver and death-dealer. The special elect, i.e., the Kohens, were also considered taboo in view of their special relation to the all-living and giving God.

lives in this manner. To my mind, it is the return, if we have ever left it, to the myth of a fixed life source and quantity. This represents a sort of pool from which life must be drawn for corporeal existence, or into which life stuff, expended in the course of living, must be returned. The *lex talionis* is then a primitive tribal rite which is but the acknowledgment of the mythic and primordial concept that there is a fixed and finite life stuff.

Those who have offended by their misuse or misappropriation of themselves while carriers of the life stuff, by the concept and demand of the majority, may be required to relinquish and give up their particular quantum of life stuff so that it may be transferred to those whom society deems more appropriate carriers or those whose promise is as yet unexpressed and unexplored.

Thus you see it is not a simple thing to take a life. Life is not taken for retribution or reprisal. There may be meaning to the concept of demonstration or example in the judicial taking of life. But more important from a mythic societal standpoint is the UR-concept of the loss or acquisition of the life stuff. That modern primitive mind, our own, still operates, as it did long ago, on the concept of exchange, acquisition, and individualism, but not social laws of the stuff of life. And simple though it may be, an execution plays out a pantomime better suited to Cro-Magnon man then to his more recent offsprings, ourselves.

Whether it be the infusing of life from the hunted caribou to the Eskimo, or the reinfusing from the elder who is destroyed to make way for the younger, from the loss due to natural causes, or civil execution, death provides a liberation of life stuff, permitting the renaissance and rejuvenation of the race. Perhaps, the Irish wake with its jubilation is a carryover of a more primitive and authentic feeling of exaltation of the death of another. The observers of Dukes' death certainly were excited and undismayed. Death provides a rebirth and rededication in its highest form, or piggish theft of life in its lowest.

Such a phrase as "The king is dead, long live the king" is an ancient formula to represent rebirth through death. When John Donne says, "Do not ask for whom the bell tolls, it tolls for thee," he means (or should mean) not simply that a part of you has died in the dying of others, but more importantly that a part has come into life or greater life through death.

A more commanding expression of the constructive principle inherent in the concept of death is immanent in the New Testament expression that "Christ died for you, He died that ye may live." Poetry, myth, fantasy or true statement, life stuff is a finite quantity.

Death imposes on the child mind of man the feeling that it gives to those who survive more than it takes away from those who "give up the ghost." This ghost so laid away returns to the common and undefilable pool for further and maybe better use. *Sic transit gloria et spiritus mundi.* So passes the glory and spirit of the world.

IX. PSYCHOTHERAPY AND THE PATIENT WITH A LIMITED LIFE-SPAN

LAWRENCE LeSHAN AND EDA LeSHAN

A patient said to her psychotherapist, "I know that I'm intelligent, I have courage, and my opinions are as good as anyone else's. Just knowing this has made a big difference in my whole life. I can see the good things I've given my children, not just the bad things. I think I even love them and my husband a lot more now." Another patient said, "You know, Doc, for the first time in my life, I like myself. I'm not half so bad a guy as I always felt I was." A shy girl had written poems all her life; they represented her ego ideal, her hopes and her dreams, but she could not believe in herself enough to let others see them. With much anxiety she showed some of them to her therapist. At his response—they were of very high caliber—she began to accept her own value as a person, and to talk hopefully about publishing her poetry. A brilliant woman with special skills in theoretical research had been blocked completely for nine years in her ability to do work in her field and was filled with self-doubt and self-dislike. One day she said with triumph and joy, "I started work on an article last night. I have it mapped out and the first two pages written. I think it's going to be pretty good." A thirty-nine-year-old woman who had never had a love relationship told her therapist one Monday morning of her wonderful weekend at the beach with a man she had met six months previously. As they had watched the sun go down, she had felt inside like the colors of the sunset. The affair begun that night was one of deep meaning to both of them, and she was able to give and receive the kind of love she had never known existed.

Each of these patients was dying from cancer. None of them lived more than one year after the reported incident, and three died within four months.

In the course of a research project into the relationships between personality and neoplastic disease, these patients and others were given the opportunity of intensive psychotherapy after their cancers had been diagnosed. Conducting over 3,500 hours of therapy with these patients brought their needs and what psychotherapy can hope to accomplish in such conditions into sharp focus.

There can be great value to the patient in the fact of someone's believing in him enough to really work to help him toward greater self-understanding and inner growth at a time when he cannot "repay" by a long period of adequate functioning—cannot "do as I tell you to and grow up to be a big, strong, successful man." His *being* is cared for unconditionally, and so he cares for it himself. The presence of the therapist affirms the importance of the here and now. Life no longer primarily seems to have the quality of something that is fading away, but takes on new meaning and validity. In the search for himself, in the adventure of overcoming his psychic handicaps and crippling, the patient may find a meaning in life that he never had found before. If the psychotherapy focuses on his strengths and positive qualities and what has blocked their full expression, rather than on pathology—as is so often unfortunately the case in psychotherapy—the patient may come more and more to value and to accept himself, and to accept his universe and his fate.

Frequently the patient who is dying has lost his cathexes, by the natural attrition of life, by inner neurotic dictates, by an attempt on his part and on the part of those closest to him to "spare" each other from discussion of their mutual knowledge, or sometimes by a partial withdrawal in a magical attempt to ease the pain of the final parting. He is, therefore, very much alone and isolated in a universe which, because of his isolation, seems hostile and uncaring—as Pascal said, "The eternal silence of these infinite spaces frightens me."[1] The therapist, by his presence and by his real interest, can give the patient meaning through warm human contact, can, by providing the opportunity for a strong cathexis, give him to anchor rope to the world and to others, so that with Bruno and Goethe, he can feel that "out of this world we cannot fall."[2] Or, like Camus's "stranger," when he had asserted, in the only way he knew, his oneness with humanity and was close to death, the patient can lay his ear "upon the benignly indifferent universe" and feel how like himself, "how warm, friendly and brotherly" it is.[3] With contact and connectedness returned, and with the focus on life rather than on death, the patient's fear of death seems to diminish considerably.

In inexorable reality situations, the fear of death—and with it guilt and self-contempt—seems usually to be related to a sense of never having lived fully in one's own way, of never having sung the unique song of one's own personality. Thus it is by the quest for one's own essence—by finding and engaging in one's own type of relationships and activities—that the fear of death may, perhaps, be most successfully eased. This view was empirically developed in this research, but it is not new; it was advanced by Montaigne,[4] and perhaps it is only a restatement of Epicurus's "Where life is, death is not."[5]

Psychotherapy, for the patient who is aware that "time's winged chariot" is hurrying him on,, cannot deal only with the technical aspects of personality as they are found in the textbooks. The larger questions are too pressing, too imminent. Values *must* be explored. As one patient put it, "Once the big questions are asked, you can't forget them. You can only ignore them as long as no one raises them." Death, the figure in the background, asks the questions, and the therapist must join in the search for answers which are meaningful to the patient. In our experience, this can be done most effectively by a search for the values most natural and syntonic to the patient—in terms of who he is, what kind of person he is, and what type of relationship would make the most sense and be the most rewarding and satisfying to him. Certainly if the patient has serious theological convictions, including some concept of afterlife, it is not the function of the therapist to attempt to disturb them; yet such convictions seldom—for who is not a child of his age?—obviate the patient's need to explore himself and his relationships with others. Thus today it is often the psychotherapist who attempts to help the person who has lost his way—and perhaps the psychotherapist also who must try to help the person who lives in the shadow of death—to find his answers to the three questions which, according to Kant, it is the endeavor of philosophy to answer: What can I know? What ought I to do? What may I hope?[6]

A common basic assumption of psychotherapy is that the psychotherapist works with a patient to increase the value of his long-term productivity and his long-term relationships with others, and, perhaps, to better his adjustment to his environment. Clearly these are not valid goals for the patient with a fatal illness. But are there other goals which therapists are committed to, or believe to be part of their responsibility? Heidegger has suggested that the age of man should not be reckoned only in terms of how long he has lived, but also of how long he has to live.[7] Within this frame of reference, it is of major importance what the person *is* and *does* during his remaining life-span—that is, what it encompasses, rather than how long it is in chronological time. Perhaps life can be seen more validly as an extension in values than as an extension in time. Here may be an approach to a philosophy of therapy that does not differentiate patients according to the length of life left to them—an evaluation which can never be more than a guess, since the universe gives no one guarantees. If a person has one hour to live and discovers himself and his life in that hour, is not this a valid and important growth? There are no deadlines on living, none on what one may do or feel so long as one is alive.

Thus our point of view in therapy is that it is important—and indeed it is all that is possible—for the therapist to help the patient at whatever point he touches the patient's life. Psychotherapy has generally taken the approach of trying to help the patient shape his life in the future, and taken the pragmatic view that results measurably in time are the only basis on which to judge success. Our view here is rather in terms of the patient's life, and respect for it, whatever its time limit.

The patient with a limited life-span has needs which psychotherapy can potentially fill. Unfortunately, however, very little therapy has been done, or is being done, with these patients. This paradox raises certain basic questions For example, one might well ask if the more than 3,500 therapy hours, out of which the material presented here was derived, should have been given to these patients. Was the work worth doing, since 22 out of 24 of them died during the course of treatment? In view of the limited number of psychotherapists available, should this time have been given instead to children or to well young adults? We are not speaking here of the *research* value of the therapy—the findings are published elsewhere[8] and must be evaluated within their own frame of reference—but of the value of the therapy in itself. Was it worthwhile? Do patients have a right to this type of care as long as they live, just as they do to physical aid? Perhaps a comparison of the approaches of clinical medicine and psychotherapy may be helpful.

In some ways, clinical medicine and psychotherapy operate according to the same rules and goals, suiting the therapeutic approach to the needs and potentialities of the patient, and having as their major goals the easing of pain and the restoration of function. However, a sharp dichotomy arises at one point. When the patient's life expectancy is clearly limited, clinical medicine does not abandon him. Although the physician may be aware that he cannot save the patient's life or restore his lost functions, he continues to attempt to soften the blow, to sustain and invigorate him, and to protect him from pain. Every medical resource is brought to bear on the situaiton. These efforts continue as long as the patient lives —and sometimes extend even to massaging the heart after the patient is technically dead!

Psychotherapy operates quite differently in this area. So long as the patient's life expectancy is not clearly limited, it may be possible for him to get psychological help. Once the termination date is dimly seen, help becomes almost unobtainable. Even if he can afford private treatment and manages to secure it, the therapist's reluctance to become involved is likely to be manifested in a quality of remoteness and detachment which is quite different from his usual therapeutic approach. This is true not only of the patient with a known fatal disease, but also frequently of those in the later decades of life. Viewing this phenomenon on a superficial level, one might come to the altogether oversimplified conclusion that the therapist's preoccupation with the patient's continued ability to function and to relate to others is greater than his preoccupation with the patient himself.

A more careful consideration of this basic difference between clinical medicine and psychotherapy may make it possible to see some of the reasons why psychotherapists, by and large, avoid working with the dying patient, and it may, perhaps, suggest some implications about the basic values and goals of psychotherapy.

There are many reasons why psychotherapists tend to feel that their task is to help the patient toward a long and healthy life. They feel that their function is not only to comfort and support—and in what denigrating terms do many psychotherapists contrast their cases in "supportive" therapy with those in "real" therapy!—but also to change him for the future. It may be worthwhile to look briefly at the reasons for this.

Each new science, as it develops, tends to exaggerate its potentialities, to see its future abilities in a somewhat magical light composed partly of hope and desire, to envision it serving as an *elixir vitae* answering mankind's greatest questions and needs. Psychotherapy is no exception—one recalls Freud's vision of answering the question of the Sphinx.[9] Psychotherapists, in working very hard to help their patients for the future as well as in the present, have often forgotten the unspoken assumption of omnipotence which is part of this orientation. Psychotherapists *cannot* mold the universe or control the future; they can help the patient *now,* in the moment in which they are in contact with him. They may perhaps need an attitude of more humility toward their own ability—one recalls someone's definition of psychotherapy as "the art of applying a science that does not yet exist"—for at present the death of patients seems to threaten the psychotherapists' basic assumption of their own omnipotence. Psychotherapy, of course, has never had any right to expect guarantees from the future. If the psychotherapist can justify his work only by the results which he assumes will appear long after he has lost contact with the patient, he had better think through his basic assumptions.

This need to help the patient in the future may be strengthened by the psychoanalytic view of the therapist as a father figure—an image which may be held not only by the patient, but by the therapist as well. As parents, therapists want their "children" to grow up and to have long, happy, mature lives. The major flaw in this orientation becomes immediately apparent if one looks at actual parent-child relationships; if a parent receives all, or a major part, of his satisfactions not from what his child is now, but from what he will become when he grows up, the relationship clearly leaves much to be desired.

Certainly it is vitally important for successful therapy that the therapist wants the very best for his patient, that he has dreams and visions for him. Only if this is true, in fact, can the patient learn to accept and value himself, to really want the best for himself. However, just as these wishes must be reality-tempered by the potentialities of the patient and his environment, they must also be tempered by the therapist's knowledge of his own realistic limitations.

Another reason for the reluctance to treat patients with a limited life-span has been suggested to us by a psychiatrist colleague. The medical man has, in his experience in medical school and in his internship, been constantly made to realize his own helplessness in the face of death. To be highly trained medically, to have at one's command all modern medical resources, and still to be unable to save a dying person can be a very heavy blow. Some of those who are most hurt by this go into psychiatry, where, theoretically, at least, death does not enter the picture. The prospect of then working with patients who will die can mobilize all of the doctor's earlier feelings of defeat and inadequacy, and arouse his resentment and resistance. In this context, remarks made by several psychiatrists about an earlier paper on the special problems and techniques involved in psychotherapeutic work with cancer patients[10] may be relevant. They did not criticize the technical concepts presented in the paper, but said that they felt the idea of intensive psychotherapy with dying patients to be "obscene" and "disgusting."

The fear of the therapist of his own hurt also seems to be a major factor in the reluctance to work with the dying patient. The feeling that a therapist develops for his patient consists of more than countertransference; there is also love and affection. When the patient dies during the process of therapy, it is a severe blow. Not only are the therapist's feelings of omnipotence damaged and his narcissism wounded, but also he has lost a person about whom he feels very deeply. It is entirely natural to wish to shield oneself from such an event, which becomes even more painful upon repetition. We believe, in fact, that a practice composed entirely or largely of patients with a limited life-span is too painful to be dealt with successfully; treating a small number of such patients seems to be a much more realistic approach.

The psychotherapist, too, cannot protect himself by the defense maneuver that necessity sometimes dictates to the purely medical specialist whose patients often die—the surgeon, for example, or the oncologist This defense—the brusque, armored manner, the uninvolved relationship, the viewing of the patient's disease as of primary interest and the concentration on its technical details to the exclusion of as much else of the person as possible—may save the physician a great deal of heartache, but it is a defense which is impossible to assume for one who is in a psychotherapeutic role. The psychotherapist's answer to the heartache must come rather from a life philosophy which regards the time left for each person as an unknown variable, and holds that the expansion of the personality, the search for the self and its meaning are valid in themselves—valid as a process, valid when they are being done, and not just in terms of future results.

These are perhaps some of the reasons why psychotherapists have done so little with patients with a limited life-span—why they have left this painful period of life to the minister, the rabbi, and the priest. To the question, What can one hope to accomplish with the dying patient?, our answer is that the validity of the process of the search for the self is in no way dependent on objective time measurements, that the expansion of the psyche—in another age, one might have called it the growth of the soul—is not relevant to the fluttering of leaves on a calendar.

Some years after his psychotherapy, a patient wrote:

> One of the primary contributions of the therapy was the certainty it has provided that I am truly alive. . . . I can recall the long years of my life and the full river of emotion that poured through me for thirty years. Surely I was alone, feeling and suffering intensely, long before the analysis began. The whole record of my life until then showed intense fear and anxiety. But there is a difference now, and I believe it consists in this: I have become integrated with life; my body, mind and psyche are intimately bound to the real world around me; no longer do I project myself almost completely into the outer world to forget myself, to avoid the inner fears, panic and uncertainty. . . . I have the firm conviction now of being really made of one piece.[11]

A sister of a patient who had died said to the therapist:

> She knew she was loved and lovable before she died. It was the first time in her life she had been able to accept this.

114

A patient's daughter wrote to the therapist:

> ... and I know that every day she grew in courage and understanding
> and was learning to fight the fears that surrounded her. With a
> woman like Mother—I suppose with any human being—an illness
> such as hers could have been the final fear to entirely hem her in and
> shut her off from human contact. But I do think that through her
> work with you, she somehow managed to win through her illness to
> greater understanding, not only of herself but of other people too.
> So please don't feel that your work was in vain. I don't believe that
> anything like that ever goes into a vacuum. Somehow it perpetuates
> itself. My father and I are changed because of the change in Mother,
> and I think it influenced her friends who visited her. Because of you,
> Mother's last months were filled with hope and thoughts of the future,
> to her very last hours. And the past few months were made far easier
> for those of us who loved her. ... Because of you, we'll always have
> a wonderful memory of Mother's last days and of the courage that
> filled them.

Of these three patients, two died during the course of therapy,
and one is still alive, years after completion. Who is to say which
of the three therapies was most worthwhile?

NOTES

1. Blaise Pascal, *The Thoughts of Blaise Pascal.* (London: J. M. Dent, 1904),
   p. 85.
2. G. Bruno, *On the Immeasurable and Countless Worlds,* quoted by H. A.
   Hoffding, *A History of Modern Philosophy* (London: Macmillan, 1900),
   p. 124.
3. Albert Camus, *The Stranger* (New York: Knopf, 1946).
4. M. E. Montaigne, *The Essays of Montaigne* (New York: Oxford University
   Press, 1941).
5. C. Bailey, *The Greek Atomists and Epicurus* (Oxford: Clarendon, 1928), p.
   401.
6. Immanuel Kant, *The Critique of Pure Reason* (Chicago: Encyclopedia Bri-
   tannica Press, 1955).
7. Martin Heidegger, *Existence and Being* (Chicago: Regnery, 1947).
8. Lawrence LeShan and Richard E. Worthington, "Some Recurrent Life History Patterns Observed in Patients with Malignant Disease," *J. Nervous and
   Mental Disease,* 124 (1956), pp. 460–465. LeShan, "A Psychosomatic Hypothesis Concerning the Etiology of Hodgkin's Disease," *Psychol. Reports,*

3 (1957), pp. 565–575. LeShan and Marthe Gassmann, "Some Observations on Psychotherapy with Patients with Neoplastic Disease," *Amer. J. Psychotherapy*, 12 (1958), pp. 723–734. LeShan, Sidney Marvin, and Olga Lyerly, "Some Evidence of a Relationship between Hodgkin's Disease and Intelligence," *AMA Arch. Gen. Psychiatry*, 1 (1959) , pp. 477–479. Le Shan, "Psychological States as Factors in the Development of Malignant Disease: A Critical Review," *J. Nat. Cancer Inst.*, 22 (1959), pp. 1–18. LeShan, "Some Methodological Problems in the Study of the Psychosomatic Aspects of Cancer," *J. General Psychol.*, 63, (1960), pp. 309–317. LeShan, "An Emotional Orientation Associated with Neoplastic Disease," *Psychiatric Quart.*, 35 (1961), pp. 314–330.

9. Ernest Jones, *The Life and Work of Sigmund Freud*, Vol. 1 (New York: Basic Books, 1953).

10. See LeShan and Gassmann, *op. cit.*

11. Jonn Knight, *The Story of My Psychoanalysis* (New York: Pocket Books, 1952), p. 201.

X. FEAR OF DEATH

NOTES ON THE ANALYSIS
OF AN OLD MAN

HANNA SEGAL

This communication is based on the analysis of a man who came to treatment at the age of seventy-three and a half and whose analysis was terminated just before his seventy-fifth birthday. He had suffered an acute psychotic breakdown when he was nearing the age of seventy-two. Following the usual psychiatric treatments (electric shocks, etc.), he settled down to a chronic psychotic state characterized by depression, hypochondria, paranoid delusions, and attacks of insane rage. Nearly two years after the beginning of his overt illness, when no improvement occurred, and when the psychiatrists in Rhodesia, where he lived, gave a hopeless prognosis, his son, who resided in London, brought him for psychoanalytical treatment.

His treatment with me lasted eighteen months. It was not, of course, a completed analysis, but it dealt sufficiently with the patient's outstanding problems to enable him to resume normal life and activity and to achieve for the first time in his life a feeling of stability and maturity. At the moment this paper is going to press, the patient has been back in Rhodesia for 18 months, enjoying good health and having resumed his business.

In his analysis I came to the conclusion that the unconscious fear of death, increasing with old age, had led to his psychotic breakdown. I believe that the same problem underlies many breakdowns in old age.

In a paper of this length I cannot give a complete picture of the patient's history or psychopathology, and I shall mention only such points as are relevant to my theme. He came from a little Ukrainian village, of an extremely poor orthodox Jewish family. His childhood was marked by fear of starvation and freezing during the long, cold winters. He had seven siblings, with nearly all of whom he was on bad terms. His mother was, to begin with, portrayed as greatly favoring his older brother, while he himself was a favorite of the father. In contrast to the mother, who was felt as cold and rejecting, the father was idolized, but also greatly feared. Following his father's death the patient, then seventeen, fled from the Ukraine, and after a long, hard struggle eventually established himself in Rhodesia as a middleman salesman. He had not tried to keep any contact with his family, which remained in the Ukraine. He also largely broke away from Jewish orthodoxy. He married and had two daughters and one son. He idealized his family but in his business relations he was suspicious and persecuted. For several years he had been addicted to secret drinking.

The circumstances of his breakdown are relevant to my theme. It became apparent early in his analysis that there were three precipitating factors of his illness. The first was his first visit to his son, who was studying medicine in London; the second was his meeting (during the same visit) his younger brother, from whom he learned that all the members of his family who had remained in Europe had perished in Hitler's camps during the war; the third and immediately precipitating factor was an incident which happened when he returned to Rhodesia. He had for several years given bribes to a man in order to get business from his firm. During the patient's absence, this man had been caught in another dishonest deal. As soon as the patient heard this, he felt terrified that his own bribery would be discovered, and within a matter of hours he was in a state of acute psychosis with delusions of reference and persecution, centering, to begin with, on his fear of his deal being discovered, and his being punished and ridiculed. He believed, for instance, that newspapers contained articles about him, that radio broadcasts were being made, people laughed at him in the streets, etc.

I suggest that my patient was unconsciously terrified of old age and death, which he perceived as a persecution and punishment; that his main defenses against this fear were splitting, idealization, and denial. His visit to London had shaken his defenses. His idealization of his only son broke down. The news he received about his family had broken down his denial of his family's death and the resulting guilt and fear of retaliation. When he returned to Rhodesia, he was faced with the fear of punishment which to him at that point represented death.

From the point of view of the patient's anxiety about death, the analysis could be divided into three phases. The first was characterized by complete denial of aging and fear of death. He described himself as having always been very young for his age, working and looking like a young man, etc., until the beginning of his illness, which he felt had robbed him of his youth and health. He unconsciously expected that his treatment would give him back his youthfulness. It soon became apparent that this denial was made possible by the patient's idealization of his son, who represented to him another self, young and ideal, into whom he had projected all his own unfulfilled hopes and ambitions. He used to send him parcels every week, and on these parcels all his interest and love centered. He put himself into these parcels sent to his son, in whom he lived, untouched by age. This relationship to his son was partly a repetition and partly a reversal of his relation to his own father. The father appeared early on in the analysis, particularly as a loving and feeding father. In relation to him the patient had developed an unconscious, intensely idealized, oral, homosexual relationship. He was the father's favorite, and he felt that so long as he had his father's love and could orally incorporate his penis, he would be protected from starvation and cold, ultimately from death. With his son he partly repeated and partly reversed this relationship. He identified himself with his father and projected himself, the favorite son, into his own son, thereby prolonging his own life. This projective identification of his young self into his son kept fears of persecution and death at bay. He also at times projected his ideal father into the son, and expected to be fed and kept alive by him forever.

Accompanying this idealization there was a great deal of split-off persecution. Parallel to his ideal son there was a son-in-law like a black twin, his main persecutor. In the past the father had been perceived mainly as loving, while the brothers were remembered for bullying and terrifying him. Any feeling of persecution that appertained to his father was immediately split off and projected onto his older brothers. In the background there was a picture of an unloving and cold mother. The feeling of persecution that he experienced in relation to her has been mainly transferred by him onto the various countries he lived in, which he completely personified, and invariably described to me as treating him badly, exploiting him, and refusing to give him a livelihood. None of this split-off persecution could, to begin with, be mobilized in the transference. I represented mainly his ideal father and son, occasionally merging with an ideal feeding mother. He had projected into me all the ideal figures, including his ideal self, in projective identification. His bad feelings and figures he had projected onto remote persecutors. So long as he could maintain this idealization of me, I would protect him from persecutors and he would be safe.

The second phase of the analysis was ushered in by the first holiday, which the patient acutely resented; when he came back it was more possible to make him aware of his feelings of deprivation. The splitting lessened; the persecution came nearer to the transference. The bad countries of the past stopped playing such a role in his analysis, and the persecution now centered on the very cold English winter which was going to kill him. Death was no longer denied, it seemed to be there, round the corner. The split between his son-in-law and his son also narrowed. To begin with, he could maintain quite simultaneously that his son brought him to London, where he was going to be made completely well again because he had his wonderful analysis, and at the same time that his son-in-law sent him to London to die of cold. Gradually it was possible to point out to him how much his son-in-law was the other aspect of his son, and how much the cold climate and country that was going to kill him was the other aspect of the analytical treatment and of myself. At that point his disappointment in his son during his first visit to London came to the fore. He had admitted that his son had not lived up to his expectations. He kept repeating: "It wasn't the same Harry, it wasn't what I meant for Harry." He admitted that he had felt completely robbed, that he had put his potency, his life, his love into his son and then that in losing the son he was losing his own potency and life and was left to face death alone. Having to face that his son, though devoted to him, led in fact a life of his own, was felt by him as losing his greatest hope, namely that his son would give him a new lease of life.

At this point it became clear to the patient that his ideal and his persecutory object were one and the same person. In the past he had split off his fear of his father onto his brothers. Now he saw clearly that it was his father's retaliation that he was afraid of. He feared that his son would leave him to his persecutors and to death and disown him, as he had left and disowned his family. Earlier on in the treatment he said that before he left the Ukraine he had to put a stone on his father, and worked very hard to earn the few shillings to purchase this stone for the grave. To begin with, it appeared as an act of mourning and piety; now it became clearer that he had to keep under the stone a very frightening and revengeful ghost of his father. In the transference it also became clear how much he had either to placate me or to control me in order to prevent me from becoming a persecutor. The persecution by his mother also came vividly to the fore: it was experienced as cold and starvation and as being abandoned or actively poisoned. He remembered that his younger brother was fed by a Christian wet nurse. One day this girl squirted some milk on his face, and he fled terrified, feeling soiled and poisoned. Being burned up or broken inside (a frequent description of his hypochondrical symptoms) was also felt by him as somehow connected with his mother. As his experiences of persecution were becoming more explicit and more connected with the real objects—myself in the transference, his son, and finally his experiences with his early family—it was also becoming clearer that these persecutions which he was either expecting or currently experiencing were felt by him as punishments. With his admission of these fears of persecution and punishment, he could overtly admit his fear of death. He felt that his idealization of me was his only protection against death. I was the source of food, love, and warmth, but equally I was the killer, since I could bring him death by withdrawing them. Idealization and placation of me alternated with only thinly veiled persecutory fears.

As this split in his perception of me lessened, so did the projection, and gradually he was able to admit his aggression in relation to me. This ushers in the third phase of his analysis, during which the persecution and idealizations gradually gave place to ambivalence, a sense of psychic reality and depressive anxieties. Slowly he was beginning to realize that, if his symptoms now appeared only during breaks and weekends, it was not simply because I, the ideal object, abandoned him to his persecutors; he was beginning to realize that everything I had given him—interpretations representing the good breast and food or the good penis—turned in my absence to bad burning, poisonous, and persecutory substances, because when he was away from me, hatred welled up in him and turned everything bad. He began to admit more freely how greedy he was for the analysis and for my presence, and how impatient and angry he was when away from me. His son and I were becoming more and more in his eyes the oedipal couple, always together when we were not with him, his son representing now the father, now his younger brother—a partner of myself standing for his mother. He recalled vividly the birth of his younger brother and the absolute fury he experienced not only in relation to the baby and the mother, but also to the father who gave mother this new baby. We reconstructed that he was weaned at the birth of this brother when he was about two. He remembered soon after that there was a fire which destroyed nearly the whole village, after which his family had been practically homeless, living in one room in an inn. It became clear that this fire was felt by him to be a result of his own urinary attacks. These were relived with such intensity that for a few nights he actually became incontinent.

We could now trace the beginning of his secret drinking to the beginning of the war in 1939, which produced in him a severe unconscious depression which he controlled by drinking. The beginning of the war unconsciously meant to him the destruction of his family. He admitted that, had he thought of it, he might have brought his family over to Rhodesia and saved their lives. He felt that he had had all the luck; he took the father's penis and then he turned against his family in anger, superiority, and contempt, and left them behind to be burned and destroyed. He unconsciously internalized them and carried inside himself the concentration camp with its burning and breaking up. But, unable to bear his depression and guilt, he split off and denied it, and turned to drink as in the past he had turned to an ideal homosexual relationship with his father. When in his analysis he began to face what the beginning of the 1939 war meant to him, he experienced a great deal of guilt in relation to his family and particularly to his mother. His previous valuation of her had become very altered. He realized what a hard struggle she had had to keep the family alive, and that the bad relations that existed between himself and her were at least partly due to the way in which he treated her, turning from her with anger and contempt to the idealized homosexual relation with his father, thereby robbing her both of himself and the father. He then experienced mourning about his family and particularly about his mother, and with it relived his early weaning situations with her, his deprivation, jealousy, envy, his urinary attacks on her which he felt had left her empty and bad, so that she was unable to feed his younger brother. Together with this changed relation to his mother and family came a very altered relation to the idea of his own death. The end of the treatment had then been already fixed, and symbolized for him his approaching death, of which he now spoke very freely. It appeared to him as a repetition of weaning, but now not so much as a retaliation and persecution, but as a reason for sorrow and mourning about the loss of something that he deeply appreciated and could now enjoy, which was life. He was mourning his life that he was going to lose, together with his analysis that was ending, and for the first time he was mourning fully the mother, and the breast that he had lost in the past. He also felt some longing for death, expressed mostly in his wish to go back to Rhodesia to meet his old friends again, which symbolized his wish to die and to meet his dead parents, of whom he was no longer frightened. But the mourning and sadness were not a clinical depression and seemed not to interfere with his enjoyment of life. In fact, he began to feel that if this life, this life-giving breast was something that he was going to mourn for so much, then, as he told me, he might as well enjoy it and do his best with it whilst he could.

In the last weeks, particularly in the last days of his analysis, he repeated some main themes in his associations, but not in symptoms, and I here select a few associations from the last week. The first day he spoke angrily about somebody who behaves like a cow; he gives one a bucket of milk and then kicks it. I interpreted that I was the cow who gave him the analysis, like the mother who gave him the breast, but by sending him away was kicking it and spoiling it all, and was myself responsible for kicking the bucket, that is my own and his death. The next day he came back to this association and said in a dejected way that it was he, in relation to his mother, who often behaved like the cow that kicked the bucket.

Later he said that she was the cow and he kicked the bucket that fed him; and he accepted my interpretation that his anxiety was that when he has to leave me he will be so angry that he will kick me inside him and spoil and spill out all the good analysis, as he felt he had done with his mother's breast, and that he would be responsible for my death inside him and for his own death. On the third day he spoke about a jug; he said that one must not judge a drink by the jug it is carried in, and he associated that he was the jug; old and unprepossessing, but the stuff that he contained could be good; it could be beer, he said, or milk. In associations it became quite clear that the beer and milk represented the good breast and the good penis, the mother and father, and myself in both roles, inside him. He felt that he had reestablished his good internal objects

At this point in his analysis he felt hopeful. He felt that his life was worth living and that, however old he was, his internal objects were rejuvenated and worth preserving. It was also clear that his children and grandchildren were no longer felt by him as projections of himself, but as his objects that he loved, and he could enjoy the thought of their living on and growing after his own death.*

Conclusions

I suggest that my patient had been unable, in his babyhood, childhood, and later on, to face his ambivalence and the resulting depressive anxiety.

He could not face the death of his object and the prospect of his own death. He protected himself against those anxieties by denial of depression, splitting, and projective identification. Those defense mechanisms, however, intensified his unconscious anxiety, in that all situations of deprivation or loss were unconsciously perceived as persecution. Idealization and denial had therefore to be intensified as a defense against both depression and persecution. When in old age he had to face the prospect of approaching death, the loss of his life appeared to him primarily as a situation of acute persecution and retaliation. He tried to counteract it by

*At this time, the patient, now in his eighties, is alive and in very good health.

intensifying mechanisms of projective identification, denial, and idealization. When his denial and idealization broke down during his visit to London, the persecution became unbearable and he became insane. The analysis of those anxieties and defense mechanisms in the transference enabled him to experience ambivalence, to mobilize the infantile depressive position and work through it sufficiently to enable him to reestablish good internal objects and to face old age and death in a more mature way.

XI. THE PROBLEM OF DEATH

HERMAN FEIFEL

Aging in the twentieth century has a singular stamp. There are more older people around than ever before because of the advances of medical science in decreasing infant mortality and prolonging life; and they enjoy better health than most of their progenitors. Nevertheless, with the shift from an agrarian to an essentially urban economy in this country, there has come a depersonalizing technology with an attendant devaluation of the older person. Traditional authority over the young, occupational status, social influence—all are becoming echoes from a dim past. The intensity of this disavowing judgment is such that even the aging person himself has become infected by its thesis. Studies increasingly reveal that many senile disorders are as attributable to the emotional deprivation and isolation visited on the aging as to their cerebral arteriosclerosis, and that sociological factors operate as insistently as disease in forwarding the admission rate of the aged into mental hospitals.

A Jewish proverb has it that "you don't need a calendar to die." Nevertheless, although it probably is true that ever since dying came into fashion life has not been safe, it is obvious that the approach of personal death is a major datum of old age. The older person's assignment is to joust not only with the possibilities of body-image changes, beleaguered hopes, the shrinkage of his social world, but with the inescapable certitude of his mortality.

For us, as psychologists, the critical question is not so much the dichotomy of life and death as how each of us relates to and copes with the cognition of oncoming extinction. A major function of practically all religious and philosophical systems of thought has been to deal with this revelation. Hegel defined history as being "what man does with death." Yet, how impoverished is our psychological knowledge in this regard. Fortunately, the *Zeitgeist* is changing. . . .

The twentieth century underlines changes not only in the significance of old age but in the interpretation of death as well. Attenuation of Pauline beliefs concerning sinfulness of the body and assurance of an afterlife has effected an accompanying diminution in people's capacity to contemplate or discuss natural death. Death no longer signals salvation and atonement as much as the threat to one's pursuit of happiness and loneliness. Fear of death no longer reveals fear of judgment as much as fear of total annihilation and loss of identity. With the waning of faith in the providential and sacred—central to much of contemporary experience—death invites our denial and hostility. Indeed, one may postulate that herein is one of the impulses of our passion for the cult of youth, and for the absurd and irrational so marked in the moral disposition of our times.

Albeit limited, because of methodological deficiencies and theoretical shortcomings, what are some of the adumbrative findings emerging from the published data presently available to us?

The import of death for older persons is multifaceted. Its specific connotations for the individual are the consequence of a commingling of factors such as one's distinctive developmental experiences, cultural context, religious regard, current life situation, capacity to meet stress, level of death threat, etc. Broadly conceptualized, two major outlooks predominate: *(a)* a materialistic or philosophic view of death as "wall" or the natural end process of life; and *(b)* a religious perspective perceiving death as the gateway to a new life. Interweaving through these two orientations are the rubrics of: (1) *calm acceptance* by those who feel relatively self-fulfilled or are anticipating a just reward; (2) *fear* or *anxious recognition* by those who behold themselves as not having captured the good life, as being stamped with a final seal of failure, or as nearer to a judgment which can punish; and (3) *resignation* by those who see themselves as having lived their term or who discern little for which to endure. Manifest also are the polarities of outright denial and wished-for consummation (Reichard, Livson, & Petersen, 1962).

The specific influence of religious outlook on the facing of personal death in older persons is not quite clear. The published data are contradictory. Some investigators (Swenson, 1961; Jeffers, Nichols, & Eisdorfer, 1961) note that religiously inclined people fear death less than do the secularly bent. Others (Faunce & Fulton, 1958; Feifel, 1959) suggest that the reverse is true. Undoubtedly, enhanced attention to the complex dimensions involved in religious commitment as well as extended methodological elegance (e.g., Allport's proper distinction between "extrinsic" and "intrinsic" religious belief) will provide us with more meaningful and consistent information.

Commanding the multiform significances of death for the individual is the cultural set of disrepute toward it. Dying and death, by and large, are evaded in the United States because many of us no longer possess the conceptual creed to encompass them meaningfully. Even when we look at death, it is through the screen of technical functions. We deal with sputtering hearts, logged lungs, distended livers—but not individuals. The death of a disease rather than of a person is our fate. The healthy and living turn their backs on death because it makes them apprehensive, if not definitely frightened.

One consequence of this state of affairs, not sufficiently heeded as yet by clinicians, is the dissembling guises which anxiety over bodily annihilation can assume. The depressed mood, fear of loss, insomnia, schizophrenic symptomatology, sundry psychosomatic disturbances—all have revealed their kinship to concerns about death. Christ (1961), Eissler (1955), and Gillespie (1963), among others, have underlined how psychiatric symptoms in the geriatric patient can mirror worry about death and its denial. Gillespie goes so far as to declare that fear of death is "the most typical traumatic factor" in fashioning senile psychosis (1963, p. 209); and incoming evidence does indicate repression of the idea of natural death in older patients. As mentioned previously, facing the prospect of death is not an exclusive "aging" problem. Nevertheless, life's finitude is both more demanding of recognition and difficult to confront, generally speaking, for the old and ill than for the young and healthy.

Consciousness of death can congeal but it can also serve as an Aristotelian *visa a tergo* impelling one toward creative performance. Though hobbled by the prevailing negativism toward death, maturity does bring along with it an appreciation of terminus which is a notable step in self-discovery. Indeed, the notion of the uniqueness and individuality of each one of us assumes full essence only in the realization that we must die. In large measure, here is the mainspring of our craving for immortality.

The paucity of psychotherapeutic work carried on with older persons is no secret. Numerous explanations are advanced for this: the elderly have "inelastic egos"; there can only be a limited return at best; and so on. Intermingled with these presumed realistic reasons is the more subtle motive of keeping aloof from "low status" individuals lest one himself become tainted (Kastenbaum, 1964). Contributing further to our therapeutic rejection of the geriatric patient, I believe, is his *memento mori* to us. Working with the schizophrenic we can think "There *but* for the grace of God . . ."; with the older person it becomes "There *with* the grace of God . . .". Sooner or later the older person forces us to look at death. Ironically, the older person wants very much to share his sentiments and thoughts about dying and death. Moreover, we are learning that dying and death are better intercepted when one feels understood by others, made to feel "in grace." The taboo we affix to death drives many of the elderly into regressive and inappropriate patterns of conduct.

In summary, aging reflects not merely a biological process but an endowed social role in which the theme of death is muffled. Our suppressive orientation toward death weighs more heavily on the older individual because of the greater immediacy of death for him. We dread death because we refuse to understand it. Ideological flight, however, does not banish death, and when death stops for us we usually find him a stranger. The heritage of a potential nuclear holocaust, among other developments, is now tending to thrust life's temporality more to the fore. Repercussions are becoming visible in our own bailiwick. Dissatisfaction is spreading with those conceptualizations, even when death is attended to, which construe attitudes toward death as inherently unfoldments of a more elemental reality (i.e., separation anxiety, although undoubtedly such clinical displacement does occur) and as essentially subordinate and derivative phenomena (i.e., from "castration fear"). Challenge is also being offered to those models of personality and psychopathology which accentuate an onerous geneticism, minimize postmaturational changes, and resort to an adhesive stimulus-equivalence outlook. The request is for more alertness to the individual's expectations, fears, hopes, dreams, goals concerning the future—and inexorable death—as well as recognition that death (and love, success, happiness) can mean different things to us at age twenty from at age sixty-five.

There is growing recognition that disregard of the intellectual and emotional predicaments arising from self-consciousness of mortality bars our access to a major gyroscope of individual and group behavior. We must establish bearings with the idea of death. Whether we do so via intelligence, love, religion—this is a matter of de gustibus. The construction of a human consciousness strong enough to admit and accept death is the charge.

As I have stressed elsewhere, I do not mean to imply that all life should be spent conquering death, or be understood as asserting that continuous facing of death is to be preferred. Man has a legitimate need to recede from death. My point is that the concept of death must be integrated into the self to subdue estrangement from the fundamental nature of our being. This should help undercut projected violence, seemingly related to compulsive needs to extrovert fear of death and killing inward alienation, and "Unheimlichkeit," and free us for more constructive experiences.

REFERENCES

CHRIST, A. E. "Attitudes Toward Death among a Group of Acute Geriatric Psychiatric Patients. J. Geront., 16 (1961), pp. 56–59.

EISSLER, K. R. The Psychiatrist and the Dying Patient. New York: International Universities Press, 1955.

FAUNCE, W. A., & FULTON, R. L. "The Sociology of Death," Soc. Forces, 36 (1958), pp. 205–209.

FEIFEL, H. "Attitudes Toward Death in Some Normal and Mentally Ill Populations," in H. Feifel (ed.), The Meaning of Death. New York: McGraw-Hill, 1959, pp. 114–130.

GILLESPIE, W. H. "Some Regressive Phenomena in Old Age," Brit. J. Med. Psychol., 36 (1963), pp. 203–209.

JEFFERS, FRANCES C., NICHOLS, C. R., & EISDORFER, C. "Attitudes of Older Persons Toward Death: A Preliminary Study, J. Geront., 16 (1961), pp. 53–56.

KASTENBAUM, R. "The Reluctant Therapist," in R. Kastenbaum (ed.), New Thoughts on Old Age. New York: Springer, 1964, pp. 139–145.

REICHARD, SUZANNE, LIVSON, FLORINE, & PETERSEN, P. G. Aging and Personality. New York: Wiley, 1962.

SWENSON, W. M. "Attitudes Toward Death in an Aged Population," J. Geront., 16 (1961), pp. 49–52.

XII. DEATH OF A PATIENT DURING PSYCHOTHERAPY

WILLIAM H. YOUNG, JR.

Little attention has been paid in psychoanalytic literature to the clinical study of the dying patient. Eissler's comprehensive study, *The Psychiatrist and the Dying Patient*,[1] brought together thinking from various fields on the subject, mainly art, literature, philosophy, and psychoanalysis, and will undoubtedly inspire further explorations. It becomes relevant, however, to consider what one means by the dying patient and whether such unique therapeutic experiences as the one I shall describe here have relevance to the mainstream of psychoanalytic work.

All of us from the moment of conception are in the process of dying, at least as far as our present knowledge takes us, whether we accept the concept of the death instinct as such or not.[2] The dying usually refers to a subgroup of the living, made up of those whose death is known to be imminent and is relatively predictable because of various concurrent events—usually a "fatal illness," or, occasionally, an external force such as a criminal or political sentence or a military assignment indicating death with no foreseeable escape.

The significant differences between the living and the dying in this sense, then, are essentially two: (1) the knowledge of the imminence of death, and its likely cause; and (2) the altered and more specific concept of the temporal span between the present and the end of life. Thus, instead of an unknown, indeterminate, and therefore easily denied or evaded eventuality, death becomes a time-limited, causally determined reality, clearly an essential and dominant part of the process of life itself. I hold with Eissler that the latter is always true, although seldom evident or fully acceptable for all of us. Hence, except for special and unusually acute features, what is true for the dying person is essentially true for all persons, and various aspects of the case that follows have definite relevance to all therapy. This suggests, too, that writing is, among other things, a way of coping with this reality and of extending one's life to deny or defeat what Eissler speaks of as the "problem of death in its full vastness and terribleness."[3]

In this case, both patient and therapist shifted back and forth between a concern with morbid fantasies and fears of the patient's death, and a concern with her death as a real and imminent prospect. These changes occurred, during the course of treatment, as shifts occurred in the diagnosis between psychological and organic illness. At the same time that I experienced these shifts and uncertainties with the patient, a series of deaths occurred among my own family and friends, the most personal of which was inadvertently revealed to the patient.

The patient was fifty-one years old at the time of referral in April 1955. Three months earlier, as she backed her car at a shopping center while her husband stood guard outside, she had suddenly, in her words, "dropped dead," falling to the seat of the car unable to move or talk. She was nauseated and later vomited. She afterwards complained to me of her discomfort at being unable "to help the boys with the stretcher" who took her to the hospital. This was typical of her approach to life—to make everyone else comfortable. While she recovered in a half hour, she was then studied thoroughly in the hospital for a week, but no evidence of organic disease was found. Psychological tests showed a Wechsler I.Q. of 138. Either conversion or cerebrovascular disease was suspected, but she was told that the attack would nor recur.

Three months later, however, while she was lying in bed, it happened again. She was rehospitalized, but organic studies were again negative. She was seen psychiatrically in the hospital, and referred, on her release, for psychiatric treatment. When she could not locate the man to whom she was referred, she frantically called around that same day and located me.

I was able to see her that afternoon and made arrangements to continue with her when I saw that she was desperate for help. She produced an enormous amount of relevant material with little prompting in that first interview, and left no doubt that she considered herself to have many problems. "Trying to grow up at fifty-one is painful," she said at the end of the first hour. "Do you think you can help?" She was tense and frightened, and described her recent attacks variously as "dropping dead," "falling through space," being "slugged from behind," or being "shot through the brain." She related numerous other somatic complaints which had been present for many years. She had, for the most part, been unaware of the fear and anger in her life, which she had defended against by a generally compliant amiability, by physical illness, and by denial.

Her devotion to her family was characterized by protectiveness and concealed deep resentments, particularly toward her brother, six years older, with whom she was closely identified. He had, at about age ten, developed a muscular dystrophy which progressed to blindness, deafness, and total helplessness before he died in 1931 at thirty-two. The patient married a man her brother's age, who agreed that she spend one month of each year with her brother. Her first baby, born the year of her brother's death and seven years after her marriage, lived only a few hours. Two other pregnancies aborted after a few months. She reacted to the baby's death with typical denial, protecting her husband and not shedding a tear. Because of her brother, she had learned early to keep her physical ailments and her negative feelings to herself and to spare her parents additional anxiety and concern.

Her highly successful professional father had died several years after her brother. Her mother, although still somewhat active at eighty-five, had had a number of strokes. Her husband had been prematurely retired, was under medical care for severe hypertension, arthritis, and gout, and was not given long to live. Because of her family's female longevity and the fact that the hospital had recently pronounced her to be in excellent health, it appeared that many years of loneliness were ahead of her, for she had no other family except an older sister and her children.

Her morbid fears and psychogenic symptoms seemed clearly related to her ambivalent death wishes, growing from this lonely prospect as well as from her long-standing identification with her father and her brother. Her relationship with her husband, although superficially compatible, had in many ways not been satisfying and had perpetuated many of her neurotic problems.

She was a vigorous, attractive, and highly verbal woman, gifted in repartee and humor, a skilled pianist, photographer, and writer. She was well read, well traveled, a keen observer and reporter, and had a remarkable capacity to plunge, however fearfully, into areas of uncomfortable and unfamiliar self-investigation. Despite her age, decision was reached quickly and collaboratively to proceed on an intensive basis to investigate the underlying causes of her acute and distressing symptoms of anxiety. She recognized their childhood origins. Since the evidence indicated that she was about to become a widow with a long and potentially productive life ahead, she seemed to be a worthwhile subject for expressive therapy.

At the end of the fourth hour, panicked by the fear that she would reveal anger, she stamped out, determined never to return. She was dissuaded from this by me and by her husband, who, fearful of his own death, was anxious that she continue. Her action, of course, revealed her anger to me, thus making accessible an important defense. She was considerably relieved when I did not respond in kind and could accept her near-violent, long-repressed affect. Her husband's subsequent interest and support was a significant strength to her throughout treatment.

To summarize an extensive case study one must of necessity select only high points. Let it be said that the patient manifested a multitude of symptoms, most of which could be explained on either psychological or organic bases. Although she had been referred directly from a complete hospital work-up, I was concerned from the outset about possible organic factors in the presenting complaints. As it turned out, these fears were groundless, but it was a symptom presumed by all to be psychological that ultimately led to the discovery of a fatal neoplasm. From the beginning, death, as both a fantasied eventuality and an ultimate reality, feared and desired, played a shifting and confusing role. Much of the time I shared the patient's confusion over whether to ignore a symptom medically and analyze it, or to see a consultant physician for medical or surgical intervention. She was constantly under the care of several doctors.

The first cancer had been clinically suspected at the hospital and was biopsied after psychiatric treatment was begun. It was a small ulcerous plaque on the tip of her nose. The patient approached the biopsy with verbal calm, but with a pulse rate of 160. Paroxysmal tachycardia had been present for years, and was one of the most useful early clues to the effectiveness of our work. In fact, it was this symptom that most clearly pointed up her need to be dealt with directly and honestly. Whenever she attempted to deny her anxiety, or when others attempted to spare her, she became irritable and shaky, and developed the telling tachycardia, which was relieved when she faced the truth, no matter how grim.

Following this biopsy, which revealed a mixed squamous and basal cell carcinoma, she received irradiation, and except for her customary set of bizarre side reactions, responded exceedingly well and was, as far as we know, cured.

Along with other problems, she made vague reference to difficulty in swallowing which went back at least seven years. Eight months prior to my first appointment, she had had complete oesophageal X-ray studies following complaints of a piece of meat having lodged in her throat. As treatment progressed, she showed steady improvement, was beginning to resume activities formerly given up, and to be more open and direct in expressing her feelings, hostile and otherwise, to her husband and to me. However, as everything else got better, the swallowing failed to yield to analysis and became gradually worse, and after several months I became definitely concerned and referred her for further X-ray studies. They revealed a large oesophageal tumor which, on biopsy, proved to be a second primary neoplasm, this time of the oesophageal mucous membrane, and the final phase of treatment had clearly begun. After having been apprised of the nature of her illness, she and her husband rejected radical surgery, which was not promising anyway, and selected further irradiation. She was told that she had about eight to ten months to live. It is of dynamic significance that the rejected surgery would have meant resection of both larynx and oesophagus for a woman whose two principal interests were talking and eating.

The period around the time of diagnosis was a crucial one for both of us. Renneker and his Chicago co-workers state, "The analyst's knowledge that an active cancer was present always produced disturbing conflicts within himself and temporarily or permanently disrupted the analytic process."[4] With this I can fully agree. It would have been easy to provoke the patient into quitting and to rationalize it as in her best interest, or to shift to bland reassurances—both common maladaptive reactions in Renneker's experience. After all, the situation was now hopeless, and analytic confrontation could become even more painful in the face of physical discomfort.

Because improvement in the handling of her emotional problems was important to both of us, there was a mutually unspoken wish that the resistant symptoms would prove other than emotionally determined, despite the tragic overtones. At the same time, serious organic illness would satisfy the patient's unconscious death wishes, still not analyzed as such, although her emotional need for physical illness had been seriously investigated. However, as Sutherland and Orbach have pointed out, ". . . patients are at least as concerned with death in surgery or with injury, and probable subsequent disruption of patterns of living as they are with the cancer itself";[5] and the task of competing with her brother's stocism, and of experiencing, his lingering dependency and discomfort, provided an additional ambivalently anticipated experience. To quote Sutherland and Orbach again, "Fears of inacceptability and of isolation can be greater sources of depression than fears of recurrence, and indeed some patients would prefer to die of cancer."[6]

My patient, then, in many ways seemed to welcome death, but was terribly afraid of invalidism and of dying. For her this problem centered clearly around her dependency struggles manifested, for example, by her initial resistance to the use of the couch; and along with the problem of honesty, the therapist was faced with that of a patient who after many months of work was showing beginning independence and now must be helped to accept without guilt or anxiety a state of dependence which one day might become as complete as had been that of her brother.

The question of honesty was decided by the patient and her husband and was the only decision compatible with our work together. She wanted to be told the whole truth, with no punches pulled.

Lael Wertenbaker, in her intimate and agonizing book about her author husband's last months with cancer, quotes him as saying, "Ever since I can remember, it had seemed to me that to be deceived about the nature of progress of serious illness, or even to suspect deceit, would go far toward destroying whatever fortitude one could summon to face one's trials."[7] This is reminiscent of Freud, who, when told that his closest colleagues and friends had almost decided not to tell him of his cancer, said, his eyes blazing, "With what right!"[8] At that, the full truth was for some time kept from him, which, Deutsch later admitted to Freud, "precluded in the future the complete confidence so essential in a doctor-patient relationship."[9]

My patient, on her return home from the oesophagoscopic examination, was weak and asked me to visit her at her home when I had the full reports and recommendations of the surgical and radiological consultants. It was, needless to say, a difficult assignment. I did not learn for some months that she had tried to make it as easy for me as possible, both out of regard for me and as a transference manifestation of her lifetime relationship with her family. From then on it was clear that false optimism brought on symptoms. She permitted me an optimistic comment only if it was based on a reality-oriented sign of improvement, or if it referred to her analytic or interpersonal perceptivity. She herself sometimes interpreted improvement as prognostically good, but unless I reminded her that recovery was unlikely, she became anxious. When I refused to let her see false hope, she would at first become angry, but this always abated shortly.

When the long and frequent trips for X-ray therapy made four hours a week difficult for her, I was faced again with a problem. I had taken great pains at the beginning of treatment to stress the importance of regularity and frequency of psychiatric interviews. How could I deemphasize this without discouraging the patient? Yet, to now demand an intensive psychiatric schedule was unrealistic and indeed cruel. Because of the physical strain and the priority of X ray at this point, we cut out one hour and planned to resume more intensive work when her schedule permitted. "Don't desert me now," she said.

X ray completed, the patient was symptomatically improved, and we resumed our previous schedule until a month before her death. The patient drove to my office herself until, at her last appointment, her right arm was too paralyzed to turn the ignition key. That night she was rushed to the hospital, where she remained calm until her death ten days later—22 months after our first appointment.

During the last several months of treatment, she was almost constantly on narcotics, which she used cautiously. Still struggling with her dependency problems, she was as concerned with the danger of addiction as with the cancer. We investigated and discussed this danger. We also discussed the progress of her symptoms and their explanations. In the last few months she developed an extremely painful and troublesome dermatitis, said to be entirely organic and coincidental (she was prone to skin disease), and even had to have some fairly extensive dental work done. Our discussions of all of these things were fruitful in themselves as we continued to search genetically and dynamically for further understanding. They also necessitated an orientation toward the future. Through the help of therapy she was able to accept her weakness and her dependency on drugs and to carry on relatively normal social relationships.

I have previously mentioned the loss of a painfully large number of people close to me in the closing months of her treatment. One of these deaths played an important part in our work. Shortly after the end of the radiation therapy, in a period of temporary and somewhat justified optimism, we were interrupted during an hour by a telephone message that my father had suffered a stroke and was not expected to live. I promptly terminated the hour, explaining simply that it was a family emergency. My father died, and I was away for a week. The patient expressed concern in my absence, and was told what had happened. In our first subsequent hour, she was again very protective of me. When I pointed out what she was doing, she was able to relate her experience at the death of her father, which had evoked protective attitudes in her toward the rest of the family. The first overt attack of nervousness had occurred on her next visit home, when an attack of tachycardia had been minimized by her mother, who suggested a trip to the World's Fair.

My experience with death and with grief outside therapy, I am sure, enabled me to better deal with my ambivalent feelings toward her impending death, and the experience helped us both to establish the "community of spirit" which Eissler has pointed out as so necessary for a successful psychotherapeutic experience in this kind of situation.[10] Her successfully protective attitude seemed to clarify the importance of mutual support in all therapy—the fact that the patient at times enables the therapist to be direct in difficult areas with the patient. It has often been observed that as the patient improves the therapist is able to be more natural and less cautious with him.

Impressive to me with this patient was something that transcends psychoanalytic terminology. Her courage was remarkable. I came to admire her and her husband greatly for their capacity to live her life to its fullest. By being willing to talk with others about her status to the extent that they were able to face it, she cleared the uncertain air, so that more interesting things could be shared. Within the limits of her physical strength, she was able to maintain contact with her many friends to the very end, despite her pain and discomfort. What Wertenbaker said of her husband— "In the perspective of death he looked closely at living and evaluated it"[11]—was true of her.

Her husband, in a letter to me a week before she died, wrote, ". . . but through it all she is calm, serene, well adjusted. For this please accept our thanks; you have given us strength to go forward." He has confirmed this feeling in a recent interview, and is himself now doing quite well.

In closing, I should like to quote Hattie Rosenthal:

> Why should a dying patient have psychotherapy when his time is so irrevocably limited? All psychotherapy is designed to help the patient cope with the contingencies of life, but in a broader sense, it is also preparation for the acceptance of death. If it makes it easier for the living to live, it can also make it easier for the dying to die. For the therapist this is a great challenge.[12]

It is significant in this case, as with Freud and Wertenbaker, that satisfaction of dependency needs was given freely and without guilt provocation, enabling the patient to reexperience something akin to a successful infancy. But there is much still to be learned about psychotherapy with the dying patient; despite the length and comprehensiveness of Eissler's book, he too leaves many things either unsaid or unexplored, and he acknowledges the need for further study. While more work in this area is beginning to appear in various medical journals, there is still only a trickle in the psychiatric and psychoanalytic press.

NOTES

1. Kurt R. Eissler, *The Psychiatrist and the Dying Patient* (New York: International Universities Press, 1955).
2. Sigmund Freud, "Beyond the Pleasure Principle," (Vol. 18, *Complete Psychological Works;* London: Hogarth, 1955), pp. 7–64.
3. Eissler, *op. cit.,* p. 295.
4. Richard E. Renneker, "Countertransference Reactions to Cancer," *Psychosomatic Med.,* 19 (1957), pp. 409–418.
5. Arthur M. Sutherland and Charles E. Orbach, "Psychological Impact of Cancer and Cancer Surgery. II: Depressive Reactions Associated with Surgery for Cancer," *Cancer,* 6 (1953), pp. 958–962.
6. *Ibid.,* p. 959.
7. Lael Wertenbacker, *Death of a Man* (New York: Random House, 1957), p. 5.
8. Ernest Jones, *The Life and Work of Sigmund Freud,* Vol. III (New York: Basic Books, 1957), p. 93.
9. *Ibid.,* p. 96.
10. Eissler, *op. cit.,* p. 246.
11. Wertenbaker, *op. cit.,* p. 16.
12. Hattie R. Rosenthal, "Psychotherapy for the Dying," *Amer. J. Psychotherapy,* 11 (1957), pp. 626–633.

XIII. DEATH AND
THE MID-LIFE CRISIS

ELLIOTT JAQUES

In the course of the development of the individual there are critical phases which have the character of change points, or periods of rapid transition. Less familiar perhaps, though nonetheless real, are the crises which occur around the age of thirty-five—which I shall term the mid-life crisis—and at full maturity around the age of sixty-five. It is the mid-life crisis with which I shall deal in this paper.

When I say that the mid-life crisis occurs around the age of thirty-five, I mean that it takes place in the middle thirties, that the process of transition runs on for some years, and that the exact period will vary among individuals. The transition is often obscured in women by the proximity of the onset of changes connected with the menopause. In the case of men, the change has from time to time been referred to as the male climacteric, because of the reduction in the intensity of sexual behavior which often occurs at that time.

Crisis in Genius

I first became aware of this period as a critical stage in development when I noticed a marked tendency toward crisis in the creative work of great men in their middle and late thirties. It is clearly expressed by Richard Church in his autobiography *The Voyage Home:*

> There seems to be a biological reason for men and women, when they reach the middle thirties, finding themselves beset with misgivings, agonizing inquiries, and a loss of zest. Is it that state which the medieval schoolmen called *accidie,* the cardinal sin of spiritual sloth? I believe it is.

This crisis may express itself in three different ways: the creative career may simply come to an end, either in a drying-up of creative work, or in actual death; the creative capacity may begin to show and express itself for the first time; or a decisive change in the quality and content of creativeness may take place.

Perhaps the most striking phenomenon is what happens to the death rate among creative artists. I had got the impression that the age of thirty-seven seemed to figure pretty prominently in the death of individuals of this category. This impression was upheld by taking a random sample of some 310 painters, composers, poets, writers, and sculptors, of undoubted greatness or of genius. The death rate shows a sudden jump between thirty-five and thirty-nine, at which period it is much above the normal death rate. The group includes Mozart, Raphael, Chopin, Rimbaud, Purcell, Baudelaire, Watteau. . . . There is then a big drop below the normal death rate between the ages of forty and forty-four, followed by a return to the the normal death-rate pattern in the late forties. The closer one keeps to genius in the sample, the more striking and clear-cut is this spiking of the death rate in mid-life.

The change in creativity which occurs during this period can be seen in the lives of countless artists. Bach, for example, was mainly an organist until his cantorship at Leipzig at thirty-eight, at which time he began his colossal achievements as a composer. Rossini's life is described in the following terms:

> His comparative silence during the period 1832–1868 (i.e. from 40 to his death at 74) makes his biography like the narrative of two lives —swift triumph, and a long life of seclusion.

Racine had 13 years of continuous success culminating in *Phèdre* at the age of thirty-eight; he then produced nothing for some twelve years. The characteristic work of Goldsmith, Constable, and Goya emerged between the ages of thirty-five and thirty-eight. By the age of forty-three Ben Jonson had produced all the plays worthy of his genius, although he lived to be sixty-four. At thirty-three Gauguin gave up his job in a bank, and by thirty-nine had established himself in his creative career as a painter. Donatello's work after thirty-nine is described by a critic as showing a marked change in style, in which he departed from the statuesque balance of his earlier work and turned to the creation of an almost instantaneous expression of life.

Goethe, between the ages of thirty-seven and thirty-nine, underwent a profound change in outlook, associated with his trip to Italy. As many of his biographers have pointed out, the importance of this journey and this period in his life cannot be exaggerated. He himself regarded it as the climax to his life. Never before had he gained such complete understanding of his genius and mission as a poet. His work then began to reflect the classical spirit of Greek tragedy and of the Renaissance.

Michelangelo carried out a series of masterpieces until he was forty: his "David" was finished at twenty-nine, the decoration of the roof of the Sistine Chapel at thirty-seven, and his "Moses" between thirty-seven and forty. During the next 15 years little is known of any artistic work. There was a creative lull until, at fifty-five, he began to work on the great Medici monument and then later on "The Last Judgment" and frescoes in the Pauline Chapel.

Let me make it clear that I am not suggesting that the careers of most creative persons either begin or end during the mid-life crisis. There are few creative geniuses who live and work into maturity, in whom the quality of greatness cannot be discerned in early adulthood in the form either of created works or of the potential for creating them: Beethoven, Shakespeare, Goethe, Couperin, Ibsen, Balzac, Voltaire, Verdi, Handel, Goya, Durer, to name but a very few at random. But there are equally few in whom a decisive change cannot be seen in the quality of their work—in whose work the effects of their having gone through a mid-life crisis cannot be discerned. The reactions range all the way from severe and dramatic crisis, to a smoother and less troubled transition—just as reactions to the phase of adolescent crisis may range from severe disturbance and breakdown to relatively ordered readjustments to mental and sexual adulthood—but the effects of the change are there to be discerned. What then are the main features of this change?

There are two features which seem to me of outstanding importance. One of these has to do with the mode of work; the second has to do with the content of the work. Let me consider each of these in turn. I shall use the phrase "early adulthood" for the pre-mid-life phase, and "mature adulthood" for the post-mid-life phase.

Change in Mode of Work

I can best describe the change in mode of work which I have in mind by describing the extreme of its manifestation. The creativity of the twenties and the early thirties tends to be a hot-from-the-fire creativity. It is intense and spontaneous, and comes out ready-made. The spontaneous effusions of Mozart, Keats, Shelley, Rimbaud are the prototype. Most of the work seems to go on unconsciously. The conscious production is rapid, the pace of creation often being dictated by the limits of the artist's capacity physically to record the words or music he is expressing.

A vivid description of early-adult type of work is given in Gittings' biography of Keats:

> Keats all this year had been living on spiritual capital. He had used and spent every experience almost as soon as it had come into his possession, every sight, person, book, emotion or thought had been converted spontaneously into poetry. Could he or any other poet have lasted at such a rate? . . . He could write no more by these methods. He realized this himself when he wished to compose as he said "without fever." He could not keep this high pulse beating and endure.

By contrast, the creativity of the late thirties and after is a sculpted creativity. The inspiration may be hot and intense. The unconscious work is no less than before. But there is a big step between the first effusion of inspiration and the finished created product. The inspiration itself may come more slowly. Even if there are sudden bursts of inspiration, they are only the beginning of the work process. The initial inspiration must first be externalized in its elemental state. Then begins the process of forming and fashioning the external product, by means of working and re-working the externalized material. I use the term "sculpting" because the nature of the sculptor's material—it is the sculptor working in stone of whom I am thinking—forces him into this kind of relationship with the product of his creative imagination. There occurs a process of interplay between unconscious intuitive work and inspiration, and the considered perception of the externally emergent creation and the reaction to it.

In her note "'A Character Trait of Freud's," Riviere (1958)

describes Freud's exhorting her in connection with some psychoanalytic idea which had occurred to her:

> Write it, write it, put it down in black and white . . . get it out, pro-
> duce it, make something of it—*outside you,* that is; give it an exist-
> ence independently of you.

This externalizing process is part of the essence of work in mature
adulthood, when, as in the case of Freud, the initially externalized
material is not itself the end product, or nearly the end product,
but is rather the starting point, the object of further working over,
modification, elaboration, sometimes for periods of years.

In distinguishing between the precipitate creativity of early
adulthood and the sculpted creativity of mature adulthood, I do
not want to give the impression of drawing a hard and fast line
between the two phases. There are of course times when a creative
person in mature adulthood will be subject to bursts of inspiration
and rapid-fire creative production. Equally there will be found
instances of mature and sculpted creative work done in early adulthood. The "David" of Michelangelo is, I think, the supreme example of the latter.

But the instances where work in early adulthood has the sculpted
and worked-over quality are rare. Sometimes, as in scientific work,
there may be the appearance of sculpted work. Young physicists
in their twenties, for example, may produce startling discoveries,
which are the result of continuous hard work and experimentation.
But these discoveries result from the application of modern theories about the structure of matter—theories which themselves have
been the product of the sculpted work of mature adulthood of such
geniuses as Thomson and Einstein.

Equally, genuinely creative work in mature adulthood may
sometimes not appear to be externally worked over and sculpted,
and yet actually be so. What seems to be rapid and unworked-over
creation is commonly the reworking of themes which have been
worked upon before, or which may have been slowly emerging
over the years in previous works. We need look no farther than the
work of Freud for a prime example of this process of books written
rapidly, which are nevertheless the coming to fruition of ideas
which have been worked upon, fashioned, reformulated, left incomplete and full of loose ends, and then reformulated once again

in a surging forward through the emergence of new ideas for over-coming previous difficulties.

The reality of the distinction comes out in the fact that certain materials are more readily applicable to the precipitate creativity of early adulthood than are others. Thus, for example, musical composition, lyrical poetry, are much more amenable to rapid creative production than are sculpting in stone or painting in oils. It is noteworthy, therefore, that whereas there are very many poets and composers who achieve greatness in early adulthood—indeed in their early twenties or their late teens—there are very few sculptors or painters in oils who do so. With oil paint and stone, the working relationship to the materials themselves is of impor-tance, and demands that the creative process should go through the stage of initial externalization and working-over of the exter-nalized product. The written word and musical notation do not of necessity have this same plastic external objective quality. They can be sculpted and worked over, but they can also readily be treated merely as a vehicle for the immediate recording of uncon-sciously articulated products which are brought forward whole and complete—or nearly so.

Quality and Content of Creativity

The change in mode of work, then, between early and mature adulthood, is a change from precipitate to sculpted creativity. Let me now consider for a moment the change in the quality and content of the creativity. The change I have in mind is the emer-gence of a tragic and philosophical content which then moves on to serenity in the creativity of mature adulthood, in contrast to a more characteristically lyrical and descriptive content to the work of early adulthood. This distinction is a commonly held one, and may perhaps be considered sufficiently self-evident to require little explication or argument. It is implied, of course, in my choice of the adjectives "early" and "mature" to qualify the two phases of adulthood which I am discussing.

The change may be seen in the more human, tragic and less fictitious and stage quality of Dickens's writing from *David Copperfield* (which he wrote at thirty-seven) onwards. It may be seen also in the transition in Shakespeare from the historical plays and comedies to the tragedies. When he was about thirty-one, in the midst of writing his lyrical comedies, he produced *Romeo and Juliet*. The great series of tragedies and Roman plays, however, began to appear a few years later; *Julius Caesar, Hamlet, Othello, King Lear,* and *Macbeth* are believed to have been written most probably between the ages of thirty-five and forty.

There are many familiar features of the change in question. Late-adolescent and early-adult idealism and optimism accompanied by split-off and projected hate, are given up and supplanted by a more contemplative pessimism. There is a shift from radical desire and impatience to a more reflective and tolerant conservatism. Beliefs in the inherent goodness of man are replaced by a recognition and acceptance of the fact that inherent goodness is accompanied by hate and destructive forces within, which contribute to man's own misery and tragedy. To the extent that hate, destruction, and death are found explicitly in early-adult creativeness, they enter in the form of the satanic or the macabre, as in Poe and in Baudelaire, and not as worked-through and resolved anxieties.

The spirit of early-adult creativeness is summed up in Shelley's *Prometheus Unbound*. In her notes on this work, Shelley's wife has written:

> The prominent feature of Shelley's theory of the destiny of the human species is that evil is not inherent in the system of the Creation, but an accident that might be expelled. . . . God made Earth and Man perfect, till he by his fall "brought death into the world, and all our woe." Shelley believed that mankind had only to will that there should be no evil in the world and there would be none. . . . He was attached to this idea with fervent enthusiasm.

This early-adult idealism is built upon the use of unconscious denial and manic defenses as normal processes of defense against two fundamental features of human life—the inevitableness of eventual death, and the existence of hate and destructive impulses inside each person. I shall try to show that the explicit recognition of these two features, and the bringing of them into focus, is the quintessence of successful weathering of the mid-life crisis and the achievement of mature adulthood.

It is when death and human destructiveness—that is to say, both death and the death instinct—are taken into account, that the quality and content of creativity change to the tragic, reflective, and philosophical. The depressive position must be worked through once again, at a qualitatively different level. The misery and despair of suffering and chaos unconsciously brought about by oneself are encountered and must be surmounted for life to be endured and for creativity to continue. Nemesis is the key, and tragedy the theme, of its recognition.

The successful outcome of mature creative work lies thus in constructive resignation both to the imperfections of men and to shortcomings in one's own work. It is this constructive resignation that then imparts serenity to life and work.

The Divine Comedy

I have taken these examples from creative genius because I believe the essence of the mid-life crisis is revealed in its most full and rounded form in the lives of the great. It will have become manifest that the crisis is a depressive crisis, in contrast to the adolescent crisis, which tends to be a paranoid-schizoid one. In adolescence, the predominant outcome of serious breakdown is schizophrenic illness; in mid-life the predominant outcome is depression, or the consequences of defense against depressive anxiety as reflected in manic defences, hypochondriasis, obsessional mechanisms, or superficiality and character deterioration. Working through the mid-life crisis calls for a re-working through of the infantile depression, but with mature insight into death and destructive impulses to be taken into account.

This theme of working through depression is magnificently expressed in *The Divine Comedy*. This masterpiece of all time was begun by Dante following his banishment from Florence at the age of thirty-seven. In the opening stanzas he creates his setting in words of great power and tremendous psychological depth. He begins:

> In the middle of the journey of our life, I came to myself within a dark wood where the straight way was lost. Ah, how hard it is to tell of that wood, savage and harsh and dense, the thought of which renews my fear. So bitter is it that death is hardly more.

These words have been variously interpreted; for example, as an allegorical reference to the entrance to Hell, or as a reflection of the poet's state of mind on being forced into exile, homeless and hungry for justice. They may, however, be interpreted at a deeper level as the opening scene of a vivid and perfect description of the emotional crisis of the mid-life phase, a crisis which would have gripped the mind and soul of the poet whatever his religious outlook, or however settled or unsettled his external affairs. The evidence for this conclusion exists in the fact that during the years of his early thirties which preceded his exile, he had already begun his transformation from the idyllic outlook of the *Vita Nuova* (age twenty-seven—twenty-nine) through a conversion to "philosophy" which he allegorized in the *Convivio,* written when he was between thirty-six and thirty-eight years of age.

Even taken quite literally, *The Divine Comedy* is a description of the poet's first full and worked-through conscious encounter with death. He is led through hell and purgatory by his master Virgil, eventually to find his own way, guided by his beloved Beatrice, into paradise. His final rapturous and mystical encounter with the being of God, represented to him in strange and abstract terms, was not mere rapture, not simply a being overwhelmed by a mystical oceanic feeling. It was a much more highly organized experience. It was expressly a vision of supreme love and knowledge, with control of impulse and of will, which promulgates the mature life of greater ease and contemplation which follows upon the working-through of primitive anxiety and guilt, and the return to the primal good object.

Dante explicitly connects his experience of greater mental integration, and the overcoming of confusion, with the early infantile relation to the primal good object. As he nears the end of the 33rd Canto of "Paradiso," the climax of his whole grand scheme, he explains:

> Now my speech will come more short even of what I remember than an infant's who yet bathes his tongue at the breast.

But the relationship with the primal good object is one in which reparation has been made, Purgatorio has been traversed, loving impulses have come into the ascendant, and the cruelty and harshness of the superego expressed in the inferno have been relieved. Bitterness has given way to composure.

In Dante, the result of this deep resolution is not the reinforcing of manic defense and denial which characterizes mystical experience fused with magic omnipotence; but rather the giving up of manic defense, and consequent strengthening of character and resolve, under the dominion of love. As Croce has observed:

> What is not found in the "Paradiso," for it is foreign to the spirit of Dante, is flight from the world, absolute refuge in God, asceticism. He does not seek to fly from the world, but to instruct it, correct it, and reform it. . . . He knew the world and its doings and passions.

Awareness of Personal Death

Although I have thus far taken my examples from the extremes of genius, my main theme is that the mid-life crisis is a reaction which not only occurs in creative genius, but manifests itself in some form in everyone. What then is the psychological nature of this reaction to the mid-life situation, and how is it to be explained?

The simple fact of the situation is the arrival at the midpoint of life. What is simple from the point of view of chronology, however, is not simple psychologically. The individual has stopped growing up, and has begun to grow old. A new set of external circumstances has to be met. The first phase of adult life has been lived. Family and occupation have become established (or ought to have become established unless the individual's adjustment has gone seriously awry); parents have grown old, and children are at the threshold of adulthood. Youth and childhood are past and gone, and demand to be mourned. The achievement of mature and independent adulthood presents itself as the main psychological task. The paradox is that of entering the prime of life, the stage of fulfillment, but at the same time the prime and fulfillment are dated. Death lies beyond.

I believe, and shall try to demonstrate, that it is this fact of the entry upon the psychological scene of the reality and inevitability of one's own eventual personal death, that is the central and crucial feature of the mid-life phase—the feature which precipitates the critical nature of the period. Death—at the conscious level—instead of being a general conception, or an event experienced in terms of the loss of someone else, becomes a personal matter, one's own death, one's own real and actual mortality. As Freud (1915) has so accurately described the matter:

> We were prepared to maintain that death was the necessary outcome of life. . . . In reality, however, we were accustomed to behave as if it

were otherwise. We displayed an unmistakable tendency to "shelve" death, to eliminate it from life. We tried to hush it up.... That is our own death, of course.... No one believes in his own death.... In the unconscious everyone is convinced of his own immortality.

This attitude toward life and death, written by Freud in another context, aptly expresses the situation which we all encounter in mid-life. The reality of one's own personal death forces itself upon our attention and can no longer so readily be shelved. A thirty-six-year-old patient, who had been in analysis for seven years and was in the course of working through a deep depressive reaction which heralded the final phase of his analysis some eighteen months later, expressed the matter with great clarity. "Up till now," he said, "life has seemed an endless upward slope, with nothing but the distant horizon in view. Now suddenly I seem to have reached the crest of the hill, and there stretching ahead is the downward slope with the end of the road in sight—far enough away it's true— but there is death observably present at the end."

From that point on this patient's plans and ambitions took on a different hue. For the first time in his life he saw his future as circumscribed. He began his adjustment to the fact that he would not be able to accomplish in the span of a single lifetime everything he had desired to do. He could achieve only a finite amount. Much would have to remain unfinished and unrealized.

This perspective on the finitude of life was accompanied by a greater solidity and robustness in his outlook, and introduced a new quality of earthly resignation. It reflected a diminishing of his unconscious wish for immortality. Such ideas are commonly lived out in terms of denial of mourning and death, or in terms of ideas of immortality, from notions of reincarnation and life after death, to notions of longevity like those expressed by the successful twenty-eight-year-old novelist who writes in his diary, "I shall be the most serious of men, and I shall live longer than any man."

Unconscious Meaning of Death

How each one reacts to the mid-life encounter with the reality of his own eventual death—whether he can face this reality, or whether he denies it—will be markedly influenced by his infantile unconscious relation to death—a relationship which depends upon the stage and nature of the working through of the infantile depressive position, as Melanie Klein discovered and vividly described (1940, 1955). Let me paraphrase her conclusions.

The infant's relation with life and death occurs in the setting of his survival being dependent on his external objects, and on the balance of power of the life and death instincts which qualify his perception of those objects and his capacity to depend upon them and use them. In the depressive position in infancy, under conditions of prevailing love, the good and bad objects can in some measure be synthesized, the ego becomes more integrated, and hope for the reestablishment of the good object is experienced; the accompanying overcoming of grief and regaining of security is the infantile equivalent of the notion of life.

Under conditions of prevailing persecution, however, the working through of the depressive position will be to a greater or lesser extent inhibited; reparation and synthesis fail; and the inner world is unconsciously felt to contain the persecuting and annihilating devoured and destroyed bad breast, the ego itself feeling in bits. The chaotic internal situation thus experienced is the infantile equivalent of the notion of death.

Ideas of immortality arise as a response to these anxieties, and as a defense against them. Unconscious fantasies of immortality are the counterpart of the infantile fantasies of the indestructible and hence immortal aspect of the idealized and bountiful primal object. These fantasies are equally as persecuting as the chaotic internal situation they are calculated to mitigate. They contain omnipotent sadistic triumph, and increase guilt and persecution as a result. And they lead to feelings of intolerable helplessness through dependence upon the perfect object which becomes demanding of an equal perfection in behavior.

Does the unconscious, then, have a conception of death? The views of Melanie Klein and those of Freud may seem not to correspond. Klein assumes an unconscious awareness of death. Freud assumes that the unconscious rejects all such awareness. Neither of these views, taken at face value, is likely to prove correct. Nor would I expect that either of their authors would hold to a literal interpretation of their views. The unconscious is not aware of death *per se*. But there are unconscious experiences akin to those which later appear in consciousness as notions of death. Let me illustrate such experiences.

A forty-seven-year-old woman patient, suffering from claustrophobia and a variety of severe psychosomatic illnesses, recounted a dream in which she was lying in a coffin. She had been sliced into small chunks, and was dead. But there was a spider's-web-thin thread of nerve running through every chunk and connected to her brain. As a result she could experience everything. She knew she was dead. She could not move or make any sound. She could only lie in the claustrophobic dark and silence of the coffin.

I have selected this particular dream because I think it typifies the unconscious fear and experience of death. It is not in fact death in the sense in which consciously we think about it, but an unconscious fantasy of immobilization and helplessness, in which the self is subject to violent fragmentation, while yet retaining the capacity to experience the persecution and torment to which it is being subjected. When these fantasies of suspended persecution and torture are of pathological intensity, they are characteristic of many mental conditions: catatonic states, stupors, phobias, obsessions, frozen anxiety, simple depression.

A Case of Denial of Death

In the early-adult phase, before the mid-life encounter with death, the full-scale re-working-through of the depressive position does not as yet necessarily arise as a part of normal development. It can be postponed. It is not a pressing issue. It can be put to one side, until circumstances demand more forcibly that it be faced.

In the ordinary course of events, life is full and active. Physiologically, full potency has been reached, and activity—social, physical, economic, sexual—is to the fore. It is a time for doing, and the doing is flavored and supported to a greater or lesser degree—depending on the emotional adjustment of the individual —by the activity and denial as part of the manic defense.

The early-adult phase is one, therefore, in which successful activity can in fact obscure or conceal the operation of strong manic defenses. But the depressive anxiety that is thus warded off will be encountered in due course. The mid-life crisis thrusts it forward with great intensity, and it can no longer be pushed aside if life is not to be impoverished.

This relationship between adjustment based upon activity in the early-adult phase, and its failure in mid-life if the infantile depressive position is not unconsciously (or consciously, in analysis) worked through again, may be illustrated in the case of a patient, Mr. N, who had led a successful life by everyday standards up to the time he came into analysis. He was an active man, a "doer." He had been successful in his career through intelligent application and hard work, was married with three children, had many good friends, and all seemed to be going very well.

The idealized content of this picture had been maintained by an active carrying on of life, without allowing time for reflection. His view was that he had not come to analysis for himself, but rather for a kind of tutorial purpose—he would bring his case history to me and we would have a clinical seminar in which we would conduct a psychoanalytic evaluation of the case material he had presented.

As might be expected, Mr. N had great difficulty in coping with ambivalence. He was unconsciously frightened of any resentment, envy, jealousy, or other hostile feelings toward me, maintaining an attitude of idealized love for me and tolerant good nature toward every attempt on my part to analyze the impulses of destructiveness, and the feelings of persecution which he was counteracting by this idealization.

When we finally did break through this inability to cope with ambivalence—indeed a pretty complete unfamiliarity with the experience—it emerged that, in all his relationships, his idealization was inevitably followed by disappointment—a disappointment arising out of failure to get the quality of love he was greedily expecting in return, and nursed by the envy of those whom he idealized.

It was out of the analysis of material of this kind that we were able to get at the reflection in the analysis of his early-adult mode of adjustment. He admitted that he was ill, and that unconscious awareness of his illness undoubtedly was the main reason for his seeking analysis. Being active, and overconcerned for others, were soporifics, to which he had become addicted. Indeed, he confessed, he had resented my analysis taking this defensive addiction away from him. He had secretly entertained ideas of stopping his analy-

154

sis "because all this thinking about myself, instead of doing things, is no good. Now I realize that I have been piling up my rage against you inside myself, like I've done with everyone else."

Thus it was that during the first year of his analysis, the patient lived out many of the techniques which had characterized his early-adult adjustment. It was with the onset of the Christmas holiday that the unconscious depressive anxiety, which was the main cause of his disturbance in mid-life, came out in full force. It is this material that illustrates the importance of the depressive position and unconscious feelings about death in relation to the mid-life crisis.

He had shown definite signs before the holiday of feelings of being abandoned, saying that not only would he not see me, but his friends were to be away as well. Three days before the end of the holiday, he telephoned me and, in a depressed and tearful voice, asked if he could come to see me. I arranged a session that same evening.

When he came to see me, he was at first afraid to lie on the couch. He said that he wanted just to talk to me, to be comforted and reassured. He then proceeded to tell me how, from the beginning of the holiday, a black gloom had settled upon him. He yearned for his mother to be alive, so that he could be with her and be held and loved by her. "I just felt completely deserted and lost," he said. "I sat for hour after hour, unable to move or to do any work. I wanted to die. My thoughts were filled with suicide. Then I became terrified of my state of mind. That's why I phoned you. I just had never conceived it as even remotely possible that I could lose my self-control like this." Things were made absolutely unbearable, he then explained, when one of his children had become nearly murderously aggressive toward his wife a few days before. His world seemed to have gone to pieces.

This material, and other associations, suggested that his wife stood for the bad aspect of his mother, and his son for the sadistic murderous part of himself. In his fear of dying, he was reexperiencing his own unconscious fantasies of tearing his mother to pieces, and he then felt abandoned and lost. As I interpreted on these lines, he interjected that the worst thing was the feeling of having gone to pieces himself. "I can't stand it," he said, "I feel as though I'm going to die."

I then recalled to him a dream he had had just before the holiday, which we had not had time to analyze, and which contained material of importance in the understanding of his infantile perception of being dead. In this dream he was a small boy sitting crying on the curb in his home town. He had dropped a bottle of milk. It lay in jagged shattered bits in the gutter. The fresh good milk ran away, dirtied by contact with the muck in the gutter. One of his associations to the dream was that he had broken the bottle by his own ineptness. It was no use moaning and crying over the spilt milk, since it was himself, after all, who had caused the damage.

I related his dream to his feeling of being abandoned by me. I was the bottle of milk—containing good milk—which he destroyed in his murderous rage because I abandoned him and went dry. He unconsciously felt the Christmas holiday as losing me, as he felt he had lost his mother and the good breast, because of his ineptness—his violence and lack of control—and his spoiling me internally with his anal muck. He then felt internally persecuted and torn to pieces by the jagged bits of the bottle, representing the breast, myself, and the analysis; as Klein (1955, p. 313) has expressed it, "The breast taken in with hatred becomes the representative of the death instinct within."

I would conclude that he had unconsciously attempted to avoid depression by paranoid-schizoid techniques of splitting and deflecting his murderous impulses away from me, through his son against his wife. These techniques had now begun to fail, however, because of previous analytical work with respect to his splitting and denial. Whereas he had been able to deny what in fact turned out to be a pretty bad situation in his home, by perceiving it merely as the product of his own projections, he now became filled with guilt, anxiety, and despair, as he began to appreciate more that in reality the relationships at home were genuinely intolerable and dangerous, and were not just a projection of his own internal chaos and confusion.

During the succeeding months, we were able to elaborate more fully his attitude toward death as an experience of going to pieces.

A connection between his phobic attitude to death and his escape into activity was manifested, for instance, in his recalling one day a slogan that had always meant so much to him—"Do or Die." But now it came to him that he had always used his own personal abbreviation of the slogan—simply "Do." The possibility of dying just did not consciously exist for him.

On one occasion he demonstrated at first hand how his fear of death had caused him always to retreat from mourning. A friend of his died. The patient was the strong and efficient one, who made all the necessary arrangements, while friends and family stood about helplessly, bathed in tears and paralyzed with sorrow. He experienced no feeling—just clear-headedness and a sense of action for the arrangements which had to be made. He had always been the same, had done the same when his father and his mother had died. More than that, however, when I interpreted his warding off of depression by means of denial of feeling and refuge in action, he recalled an event which revealed the unconscious chaos and confusion stirred within him by death. He remembered how, when a cousin of his had suddenly collapsed and died a few years before, he had run back and forth from the body to the telephone to call for a doctor, oblivious of the fact that a small group of people had gathered about the body, and not realizing that everyone but himself was perfectly aware that his cousin was quite dead, and had been for some time before he arrived upon the scene.

The chaos and confusion in the patient in connection with death, I would ascribe to his unconscious infantile fantasies equivalent to death—the fantasies of the destroyed and persecuting breast, and of his ego being cut to pieces.

Mainly, I think, because of the love he got from his father, probably reinforcing his own innate good impulses and what he has had described to him as good breast-feeding in the first five weeks with his mother, he had been able to achieve a partial working through of the infantile depressive position, and to develop his good intellectual capacities. The partial character of his working through was shown in the extent of his manic denial and activity, and his excessive use of splitting, introjection and projection, and projective and introjective identification.

During the period of early adulthood—the twenties and early thirties—the paranoid-schizoid and manic-defense techniques were sufficiently effective. By means of his apparent general success and obsessional generosity, he was able to live out the role of the good mother established within, to nurture the good part of himself projected into others, to deny the real situation of envy and greed and destructiveness expressed by him as his noxiousness, and to deny the real impoverishment of his emotional life, and lack of genuine love and affection in his behavior as both husband and father.

With the onset of mature adulthood in his mid-thirties, his defensive techniques began to lose their potency. He had lost his youth, and the prospect of middle age and of eventual death stimulated a repetition and a re-working-through of the infantile depressive position. The unconscious feelings of persecution and annihilation which death represented to him were reawakened.

He had lost his youth. And with both his parents dead, nobody now stood between himself and the grave. On the contrary, he had become the barrier between his children and their perception of death. Acceptance of these facts required constructive resignation and detachment. Unconsciously such an outlook requires the capacity to maintain the internal good object, and to achieve a resigned attitude to shortcomings and destructive impulses in oneself, and imperfections in the internal good object. My patient's unconscious fantasies of intolerable noxiousness, his anxieties of having polluted and destroyed his good primal object so that he was lost and abandoned and belonged nowhere, and his unconscious fantasies of the badness of his internalized mother as well as his father, precluded such detachment and resignation. The psychological defenses which had supported his adjustment in early-adult life—an adjustment of a limited kind, of course, with a great core of emotional impoverishment—failed him at the mid-life period when, to the persecutory world in which he unconsciously lived, were added his anxieties about impending middle and old age, and death. If he had had a less well-established good internal object, and had been innately less constructive and loving, he might have continued his mature adult life along lines similar to his early-adult type of adjustment; but if he had, I think his mid-life crisis would have been the beginning of a deterioration in his character, and bouts of depression and psychosomatic illness, due to the depth and chronicity of his denial and self-deception, and his distorted view of external reality.

As it has worked out, however, the positive factors in his personality make-up enabled him to utilize his analysis, for which he developed a deep sense of value and appreciation. The overcoming of splitting and fragmentation first began to show in a session in which, as out of nowhere, he saw two jagged-edged right-angled triangles. They moved together, and joined to make a perfect square. I recalled the dream with the broken bits of bottle to him. He replied, "It's odd you should mention that; I was just thinking of it. It feels like the bits of glass are coming together."

Evasion of Awareness of Death

One case history does not of course prove a general thesis. It can only illustrate a theme, and the theme in this instance is the notion that the circumstances met by this patient at the mid-life phase are representative of a general pattern of psychological change at this stage of life. The extent to which these changes are tied up with physiological changes is a question I am not able to tackle. One can readily conjecture, however, that the connection must be an important one—libido, the life-creating impulse, represented in sexual drive, is diminishing, and the death instinct is coming relatively more into the ascendant.

The sense of the agedness of parents, coupled with the maturing of children into adults, contributes strongly to the sense of aging— the sense that it is one's own turn next to grow old and die. This feeling about the age of parents is very strong—even in patients whose parents died years before there is the awareness at the mid-life period that their parents would then have been reaching old age.

In the early-adult phase of life, contemplativeness, detachment, and resignation are not essential components of pleasure, enjoyment and success. Manically determined activity and warding off of depression may therefore—as in the case of Mr. N—lead to a limited success and pleasure. Splitting and projection techniques can find expression in what are regarded as perfectly normal patterns of passionate support for idealized causes, and equally passionate opposition to whatever may be felt as bad or reactionary.

With the awareness of the onset of the last half of life, unconscious depressive anxieties are aroused, and the repetition and continuation of the working-through of the infantile depressive position are required. Just as in infancy—to quote Klein again

(1940, p. 314)—"satisfactory relations to people depend upon the
infants having succeeded against the chaos inside him (the depressive position) and having securely established his 'good' internal
objects," so in mid-life the establishment of a satisfactory adjustment to the conscious contemplation of one's own death depends
upon the same process, for otherwise death itself is equated with
the depressive chaos, confusion, and persecution, as it was in
infancy.

When the prevailing balance between love and hate tends more
toward the side of hate, when there is instinctual defusion, there
is an overspill of destructiveness in any or all of its various forms—
self-destruction, envy, grandiose omnipotence, cruelty, narcissism,
greed—and the world is seen as having these persecuting qualities
as well. Love and hate are split apart; destruction is no longer
mitigated by tenderness. There is little or no protection from
catastrophic unconscious fantasies of annihilating one's good objects. Reparation and sublimation, the processes which underly
creativeness, are inhibited and fail. And in the deep unconscious
world there is a gruesome sense of invasion and habitation by the
psychic objects which have been annihilated.

In primitive terms, the process of sculpting is experienced partly
as a projective identification, in which the fear of dying is split off
and projected into the created object (representing the creative
breast) . Under the dominance of destructiveness the created object,
like the breast, is felt to

> remove the good or valuable element in the fear of dying, and to
> force the worthless residue back into the infant. The infant who
> started with a fear that he was dying ends up by containing a name-
> less dread [Bion, 1962].

The conception of death is denuded of its meaning, and the process
of sculpted creativity is stopped. It is the experience of a patient
who, having created a work of art by spontaneous effusion, found
that "it goes dead on me; I don't want to have anything more to
do with it; I can never work on it further once it is outside, so I can
never refine it; it completely loses its meaning for me—it's like a
strange and foreign thing that has nothing to do with me."

The ensuing inner chaos and despair is unconsciously fantasied
in terms akin to an inferno: "I came to myself within a dark wood

. . . savage and harsh and dense." If this state of mind is not surmounted, hate and death must be denied, pushed aside, warded off,
rejected. They are replaced by unconscious fantasies of omnipotence, magic immortality, religious mysticism, the counterpart of
infant fantasies of being indestructible and under the protective
care of some idealized and bountiful figure.

A person who reaches mid-life, either without having successfully
established himself in marital and occupational life, or having
established himself by means of manic activity and denial with
consequent emotional impoverishment, is badly prepared for
meeting the demands of middle age, and getting enjoyment out
of his maturity. In such cases, the mid-life crisis, and the adult
encounter with the conception of life to be lived in the setting of
an approaching personal death, will likely be experienced as a
period of psychological disturbance and depressive breakdown.
Or breakdown may be avoided by means of a strengthening of
manic defenses, with a warding off of depression and persecution
about aging and death, but with an accumulation of persecutory
anxiety to be faced when the inevitability of aging and death
eventually demands recognition.

The compulsive attempts, in many men and women reaching
middle age, to remain young, the hypochondriacal concern over
health and appearance, the emergence of sexual promiscuity in
order to prove youth and potency, the hollowness and lack of
genuine enjoyment of life, and the frequency of religious concern,
are familiar patterns. They are attempts at a race against time.
And in addition to the impoverishment of emotional life contained
in the foregoing activities, real character deterioration is always
possible. Retreat from psychic reality encourages intellectual dis-
honesty, and a weakening of moral fiber and of courage. Increase
in arrogance, and ruthlessness concealing pangs of envy—or self-
effacing humbleness and weakness concealing fantasies of omnipotence—are symptomatic of such change.

These defensive fantasies are equally as persecuting, however,
as the chaotic and hopeless internal situation they are meant to
mitigate. They lead to attempts at easy success, at a continuation
on a false note of the early-adult lyricism and precipitate creation
—that is, creation which, by avoiding contemplation, now seeks
not to express but to avoid contact with the infantile experience

of hate and of death. Instead of creative enhancement by the intro-
duction of the genuinely tragic, there is emotional impoverishment
—a recoil away from creative development. As Freud incisively
remarked: "Life loses in interest, when the highest stake in the
game, life itself, may not be risked." Here is the Achilles heel of
much young genius.

Working Through the Depressive Position

When, by contrast, the prevailing balance between love and hate
is on the side of love, there is instinctual fusion, in which hate can
be mitigated by love, and the mid-life encounter with death and
hate takes on a different hue. Revived are the deep unconscious
memories of hate, not denied but mitigated by love; of death and
destruction mitigated by reparation and the will to life; of good
things injured and damaged by hate, revived again and healed by
loving grief; of spoiling envy mitigated by admiration and by grati-
tude; of confidence and hope, not through denial, but through the
deep inner sense that the torment of grief and loss, of guilt and
persecution, can be endured and overcome if faced by loving
reparation.

Under constructive circumstances, the created object in mid-life
is experienced unconsciously in terms of the good breast which
would in Bion's (1962) terms

> moderate the fear component in the fear of dying that had been pro-
> jected into it and the infant in due course would re-introject a now
> tolerable and consequently growth-stimulating part of its personality.

In the sculpting mode of work the externally created object,
instead of being experienced as having impoverished the personality, is unconsciously reintrojected, and stimulates further unconscious creativeness. The created object is experienced as life-giving.
The transformation of the fear component in the fear of dying
into a constructive experience is forwarded. The thought of death
can be carried in thinking, and not predominantly in projective
identification, so that the conception of death can begin to find its
conscious realization. The reality-testing of death can be carried
out in thinking, separated partly from the process of creating an
external object. At the same time the continuing partial identification of the creative sculpting with the projection and reintrojection

of the fear of dying gives a stimulus to the sculpting process because of its success in forwarding the working through of the infantile projective identification with a good breast.

Thus in mid-life we are able to encounter the onset of the tragedy of personal death with the sense of grief appropriate to it. We can live with it, without an overwhelming sense of persecution. The infantile depressive position can be further worked through unconsciously, supported by the greater strength of reality-testing available to the nearly mature individual. In so reworking through the depressive position, we unconsciously regain the primitive sense of wholeness—of the goodness of ourselves and of our objects —a goodness which is sufficient but not idealized, not subject to hollow perfection. The consequent feeling of limited but reliable security is the equivalent of the infantile notion of life.

These more balanced conditions do not, however, presuppose an easy passage through the mid-life crisis. It is essentially a period of purgatory—of anguish and depression. So speaks Virgil:

> Down to Avernus the descent is light. But thence thy journey to re-trace, there lies the labor, there the mighty toil by few achieved.

Working through again the infantile experience of loss and of grief, gives an increase in confidence in one's capacity to love and mourn what has been lost and what is past, rather than to hate and feel persecuted by it. We can begin to mourn our own eventual death. Creativeness takes on new depths and shades of feeling. There is the possibility, however, of furthering the resolution of the depressive position at a much deeper level. Such a working through is possible if the primal object is sufficiently well established in its own right and neither excessively idealized nor devalued. Under such circumstances there is a minimum of infantile dependence upon the good object, and a detachment which allows confidence and hope to be established, security in the preservation and development of the ego, a capacity to tolerate one's shortcomings and destructiveness, and withal, the possibility of enjoyment of mature adult life and old age.

Given such an internal situation, the last half of life can be lived with conscious knowledge of eventual death, and acceptance of this knowledge, as an integral part of living. Mourning for the dead self can begin, alongside the mourning and reestablishment of the lost objects and the lost childhood and youth. The sense of life's continuity may be strengthened. The gain is in the deepening of awareness, understanding and self-realization. Genuine values can be cultivated—of wisdom, fortitude and courage, deeper capacity for love and affection and human insight, and hopefulness and enjoyment—qualities whose genuineness stems from integration based upon the more immediate and self-conscious awareness and acceptance not only of one's own shortcomings but of one's destructive impulses, and from the greater capacity for sublimation which accompanies true resignation and detachment.

Sculpted Creativity

Out of the working through of the depressive position, there is further strengthening of the capacity to accept and tolerate conflict and ambivalence. One's work need no longer be experienced as perfect. It can be worked and reworked, but it will be accepted as having shortcomings. The sculpting process can be carried on far enough so that the work is good enough. There is no need for obsessional attempts at perfection, because inevitable imperfection is no longer felt as bitter persecuting failure. Out of this mature resignation comes the serenity in the work of genius, true serenity, serenity which transcends imperfection by accepting it.

Because of the greater integration within the internal world, and a deepening of the sense of reality, a freer interaction can occur between the internal and the external worlds. Sculpted creativity expresses this freedom with its flow of inspiration from inside to outside and back, constantly repeated, again, and yet again. There is a quality of depth in mature creativity which stems from constructive resignation and detachment. Death is not infantile persecution and chaos. Life and the world go on, and we can live on in our children, our loved objects, our works, if not in immortality.

The sculpting process in creativity is facilitated because the preparation for the final phase in reality-testing has begun—the reality-testing of the end of life. For everyone, the oncoming years of the forties are the years when new starts are coming to an end. This feeling can be observed to arise in a particularly poignant way by the mid-forties. This sense of there being no more changing is anticipated in the mid-life crisis. What is begun has to be finished. Important things that the individual would have liked to achieve, would have desired to become, would have longed to have, will not be realized. The awareness of oncoming frustration is especially intense. That is why, for example, the issue of resignation is of such importance. It is resignation in the sense of conscious and unconscious acceptance of inevitable frustration on the grand scale of life as a whole.

This reality-testing is the more severe the greater is the creative ability of the individual, for the time scale of creative work increases dramatically with ability. Thus the experience is particularly painful in genius, capable of achieving vastly more than it is possible to achieve in the remaining years, and therefore frustrated by the immense vision of things to be done which will not be done. And because the route forward has become a cul de sac, attention begins its Proustian process of turning to the past, working it over consciously in the present, and weaving it into the concretely limited future. This consonance of past and present is a feature of much mature adult sculpting work.

The positive creativeness and the tone of serenity which accompany the successful endurance of this frustration, are characteristic of the mature production of Beethoven, Goethe, Virgil, Dante, and other giants. It is the spirit of the "Paradiso," which ends in words of strong and quiet confidence:

> But now my desire and will, like a wheel that spins with even motion, were resolved by the Love that moves the sun and other stars.

It is this spirit, on a smaller scale, which overcomes the crisis of middle life, and lives through to the enjoyment of mature creativeness and work in full awareness of death which lies beyond—resigned but not defeated. It is a spirit that is one criterion of the successful working through of the depressive position in psychoanalysis.

REFERENCES

BION, W. (1962). *Learning from Experience*. London: Heinemann; New York: Basic Books.

FREUD, S. (1915). "Thoughts for the Times on War and Death." Vol. 14, *The Standard Edition of the Complete Psychological Works of Sigmund Freud*. London: Hogarth, 1955.

KLEIN, M. (1935). "A Contribution to the Psychogenesis of Manic-Depressive States." In *Contributions to Psycho-Analysis*. London: Hogarth, 1948.

———(1940). "Mourning and Its Relation to Manic-Depressive States." In *Contributions to Psychoanalysis*. London: Hogarth, 1948.

———(1955). "On Identification." In *New Directions in Psycho-Analysis*. London. Tavistock; New York: Basic Books.

RIVIERE, J. (1958). "A Character Trait of Freud's." In *Psycho-Analysis and Contemporary Thought*. Edited by J. D. Sutherland. London: Hogarth.

XIV. THE FEAR OF DEATH
AS AN INDISPENSABLE FACTOR
IN PSYCHOTHERAPY

HATTIE R. ROSENTHAL

The one irrefutable fact of life is death. It is an inescapable reality for man, "who knows that at some future moment he will not be ... who is always in a dialectical relation with non-being, death" (1, p. 42).

Inescapable reality though death may be, it provokes profound reactions in the human personality. Adler, citing "typical occasions for the onset of neurosis," listed among them "mortal danger"— imminent fear of death (2). Horney has commented that we must accept the existence of anxiety in the face of death (3). Greenberg and Alexander see death anxiety as "an intrinsic part of human life." (4).

Having elaborated on "Psychotherapy for the Dying" (5), this writer felt motivated to direct her therapeutic interest further, toward the significance of the fear of death in any human being regardless of age, health, sex, environment, or culture. This discussion will be limited to the Western culture in which we live, as the death concept of Eastern culture differs fundamentally from ours.

We seem too easily to overcome the fear of death immanent in our patients, unless we very consciously and conscientiously scrutinize this specific fear, which hides behind many other fears, anxieties, and phobias. Kingman has described a number of common phobias and concluded that one universal fear—the fear of death—is rooted in all of them, the phobias serving as compensatory mechanisms (6). According to Zilboorg, "no one is free of the fear of death. ... That this fear is prominent in a number of psychopathological conditions every psychiatrist knows. The anxiety

166

neuroses, the various phobic states, even a considerable number of depressive suicidal states and many schizophrenias amply demonstrate the ever-present fear of death which becomes woven into the major conflicts of the given psychopathological conditions" (7).

Therapists frequently understand a phobia as a covering-up of a socially or morally unacceptable demand and may overlook the fact that underlying the psychodynamics of the phobia, is, in its ultimate analysis, the wish to die. "Death . . . is, in part, desired and sought by all. But dying, that is, corruption, means leave-taking, loss, surrender, and sacrifice, and most of us try to escape" (8). The wish to die may thus cause the fear of dying. An example may illustrate this concept.

> A patient named Anne suffered from a severe claustrophobia. Underlying this phobia was her demand for freedom, which she felt she had lost by marrying. Extensive conversations during her therapy produced in Anne more confidence in the regaining of her lost freedom. It was to be expected, in the light of this development, that the claustrophobia would be dissolved. Contrary to the expectation of both therapist and patient in this regard, the phobia condition recurred after two weeks of remission. This drove the patient to feel "half crazy."

Either our discovery had not been the curative agent, and we were on the wrong track, or the discovery had not gone deep enough to provide a cure. We returned to our original assumption of the deprivation of freedom by marriage, and went on to discuss her concept of freedom and of non-freedom at length. What, the therapist asked, was the ultimate deprivation of freedom in the patient's opinion? To which she spontaneously answered, "Death." Did she remember whether she had ever wished to die? Yes, this had been for quite a while a conscious wish, though at the same time she was horrified at the thought of her own death. Could her fear of narrow, closed rooms (elevators) indicate her fear of the grave or the coffin? Such discussion led to considerable relief, and shortly afterward the patient's symptoms vanished.

Literature on the Death Fear

There is an amazing paucity of material in the literature on the psychotherapeutic handling of the death fear. Wahl has written:

"The fear of death, or specific anxiety about it, has almost no description in the psychiatric literature" (9). This lack has been mentioned obliquely by Aronson and associates as follows: "Death has been a consistently untouchable area for study and research. Primitive taboos against touching the dead body seem to have carried over even into civilized intellectual pursuits on the subject. One manifestation of this is a dearth of published material in this area" (10). Truly, the thought of death is so unpleasant that avoidance of it extends even to psychoanalytic literature and investigation. Psychotherapists themselves may harbor such unrecognized fear, which causes them unconsciously to avoid the subject as much as possible.

Freud stated unequivocally that "the aim of all life is death," and firmly assumed the existence of "the ego or death instincts" in opposition to "sexual or life instincts" (11). Early psychoanalytic writings did little more than discuss and debate Freud's postulations. While some attention has been given to the death fear, rather than the death instinct, in modern psychologic and psychoanalytic literature little if any mention has been made of the need to bring this all-encompassing inner agent of neurosis into the open in psychotherapy. Unlimited attention, on the other hand, has been given to studying the psychotherapeutic treatment of all other instincts, impulses, thoughts, preoccupations, feelings, and experiences, which in many cases are actually manifestations of the underlying fear of death. Often, perhaps always, "anxiety concerning death may mask other areas of conflict, such as oedipal or aggressive problems . . . conversely, other areas of manifest anxiety may conceal death anxiety" (4).

Williams, discussing fear of death, points out "the difference in approach to these patients before and after the fear of death reaches consciousness . . ." and states: "I assume that the aim of treatment is to work towards the secret wish for death, and then to look at it with the patient in all its horror and beauty, thus peopling the void with images from which new possibilities of life may spring" (12). This writer agrees with Williams, but wishes to emphasize that the therapist cannot leave this reaching of consciousness to chance. Examination of this fear is necessary in every analysis; it is the therapist's responsibility to be aware of this fear and to *help* the patient uncover it. In mentioning the pitfalls in the countertransference in connection with the fear of death, Williams fails to cite the analyst's own fear, which has perhaps not been overcome.

Zilboorg states: "The fear of death, simple and natural though it appears, requires considerable analysis in order to be understood. If we are to comprehend a little of the world about us, it is imperative that we gain as much understanding as is possible of the complexity of this fear" (7). Surely there is no better way to analyze this fear than to study it specifically, with and in our patients, rather than as a theoretical intellectual exercise.

Zilboorg points out the human need to repress the fear of death. "If this fear were constantly conscious, we should be unable to function normally. It must be properly repressed to keep us living with any modicum of comfort. . . . We know very well that to repress . . . means too that every now and then we automatically open some psychological safety valve and gradually let out some of the tension, in order to avoid accumulating too much of it" (7). In the context of the present paper, these statements further illustrate this writer's contention that the fear of death *must* enter into every psychoanalysis. Whether deeply repressed, or being discharged occasionally in various direct or oblique manifestations, it exists in every individual and it must be dealt with and understood. If thoughts and fears of death are left alone, they slide back, into the unconscious, and from there they operate as unseen enemies attacking from ambush.

Many papers and studies could be cited, each touching on the fear of death, each a contribution which must lead us inevitably to acknowledgment of the universality of this fear. This point has perhaps been sufficiently made. But one further point, this writer feels, cannot be too greatly stressed: namely, that so universal and basic a fear must be considered in every psychotherapeutic treatment. Without such consideration, treatment cannot fully plumb the depths of psychoneurotic or psychopathologic manifestations.

"Since Freud has made death a central concept of his psychological system," Eissler wrote, "one would have expected that psychoanalysts would devote more effort to the study of death itself. Strangely enough this has not happened" (13, p. 39). Eissler stressed "the supreme effort to deny death . . . characteristic of present American civilization" (13, p. 45). His remark on our "supreme effort to deny death" is an astute observation. Its reverse, a concentrated effort to understand rather than to deny, should be the watchword of every psychotherapist.

Therapy

Once we have given recognition to the almost universal fear of death, we must discuss with every patient his concept of death. The opportunity will present itself in one form or another, be it expressed in dreams, in occasional remarks, or even by jokes. (One patient flippantly said: "I will either commit suicide or go to Florida, just to get away!") Were the therapist to avoid getting down to a discussion about death, he would be cooperating with the patient's own taboo, and would thus be supportive of the death anxiety rather than instrumental in breaking it down. This omission could interfere with and even jeopardize the eventual therapeutic success.

Some patients have expressed themselves strongly on the subject to this writer. They have stated that an open and honest discussion of death and dying has liberated them from heretofore unrecognized chains. Fearing death less enabled them to relate more positively to life.

The patient welcomes the opportunity to talk about his fears to the therapist. He is curious to know what the therapist's reaction is to death. He hopes the therapist can supply the "answers" that he has not found by himself or through others. He in some way expects the therapist to provide him with some satisfactory solution to the questing search through which he hopes in some measure to offset the fear of death. If this phenomenon is dealt with in an intelligent and honest fashion, the patient is encouraged to face and accept death as the end of life, and to conquer his surplus of fear, the neurotic evidence of his quandary.

> A forty-two-year-old patient who knew he had a fatal illness, began to suffer unbearable attacks of convulsions which, according to the treating physicians, were not connected with the disease. Interpretation of a dream brought to light his lack of reconciliation to the idea of death, and the fear which gripped him. The convulsions were life (motion) kicking away death, seen as a man in a black mask. The patient realized from the discussion of the dream that he could not fight death, and thereafter found peace. The convulsions disappeared.

Self-protection

One may question whence stems the fear of death in an individual who has not been in any particular contact with death. By the same token one might well ask whence all our feelings stem! Are we not born with elementary feelngs, of which some develop and some remain latent? These elementary feelings are provided by Nature as protective devices. Some may never be developed or recognized because the events for which they would produce preventive reactions may not occur.

Certainly one may question why the fear of death, in particular, is so basic to the human personality as to be considered an almost universal phenomenon. The answer appears to be as simple as it is logical. Death is inevitable, a certainty which all mortals face. As Voltaire wrote, "The human race is the only one that knows it must die." However, although we know that death is inevitable, we are usually not confronted with this absolute certainty. Still, the fear of inevitable death permanently underlies life. This fear must be discovered. The therapist has to be on a constant lookout to detect the many ramifications of the death fear which have heretofore gone unrecognized.

Other factors of human life are less predictable than the immanence of death, the one sure event in every life. It would appear that Nature has equipped us with the fear of death as a specifically strong feeling which is developed in everyone. This fear causes us to push the eventuality of actual death as far as possible into the future. The further we push it away, because of our fear, the less it seems acutely threatening. Thus, the normal fear of death is actually a self-protective mechanism.

Death as a Cutting-off

In his article "Fear of Death" (14), Howard refers to Freud's position as follows: "He [Freud] regarded it [the fear of death] purely as a secondary substitutive phenomenon of the castration fear which grew out of an inadequately resolved Oedipal conflict."

If one can accept the belief that the fear of death stems from the castration fear, which in turn grows out of an inadequately resolved oedipal conflict, why not then accept the converse—that the castration fear stems from the much more basic, original fear of death?

The classic castration fear is concentrated on loss of a member, a portion of the whole. The fear of death is concerned with the threat of destruction not of a part, but of the whole being. Implicit here is the concept of death as a cutting-off, an extension of castration that includes the whole physical and psychologic being.

Castration is partial loss, death is loss in its totality—everything is cut off. Is it not then feasible that the death-fearer, in his frantic denial of the ultimate cutting-off of his entire being, in his inability to contemplate with any kind of equanimity his own passing, substitutes for the fear of death a secondary fear—namely, that of the partial loss which he would suffer through castration?

Suicide as Power

There is a wry joke about a man who was so afraid of death that he killed himself. Perhaps behind this joke (as behind all jokes) lies a truth. The fear of death may have become so overwhelming in this man that it was intolerable. He therefore escaped a prolongation of this fear by bringing about the one condition that could end it— death. This anxious individual may have had another motive in mind when he committed suicide instead of awaiting his death, which may be explainable in terms of Adler's "lust for power" concept (15).

As Fromm-Reichmann has said, "The fact that time and cause of death are unpredictable conveys a painful sense of ultimate powerlessness" (16, p. 313). This "powerlessness" is the unbearable factor for the individual who takes the power into his own hands by the act of suicide. Consequently, suicide may be looked at partially as a power maneuver in the Adlerian sense, which counteracts a fear of becoming overpowered.

One may surmise that the fear of being overpowered springs from the fear originally felt by the child toward the giant parents in whose hands lay the power to command and direct the child's life. The parents can put the child into a bright room (life), or close him up in a dark room (death). Thus, dark is for the child identical with punishment and death.

Fear of the Unknown

The fear of the unknown was revealed by a patient who first gave the diagnostic impression of schizophrenic reaction of the catatonic type. Her pseudo-catatonia, as it proved to be, was a stratagem to provide her with "rehearsals" of the death experience, in an attempt to alleviate her fear of death, the unknown. Her condition was characterized by stupor and a mutist appearance, which she may have produced in an autohypnotic way.

Fear of Punishment

The fear of punishment is a universal and usually a normal reaction (lacking in the sociopathic personality). In the neurotic personality this fear may be so exaggerated as to become intolerable. Again, the fear of death is the ultra-reaction to the fear of punishment.

The dream of a young woman of twenty-seven gives us some information about the connection between death anxiety and fear of punishment:

> Our family name is written in oversized letters on a tombstone. My husband and I are compelled to stand in front of it and face it. I have the shivers, but I cannot move away.

This patient had had an abortion, and felt that her entire family should be extinguished as atonement. She thought of impending death as "lethal punishment" for the abortion crime, and the death-punishment anxiety pursued her day and night.

Another patient, given to superstition, was tortured by the fear that evil spirits begrudged him his life. "The evil spirits are envious," he would say. In therapy he discovered his own envy, which he had externalized. He then recognized that the "evil spirits" who "chased him into death" were his self-devised death-punishments for his own "sinful envy."

Loneliness

The human being is a *zoon politikon* (Gr.: a social being). One of his fundamental needs is to relate to other human beings. It is this need for intimacy which Sullivan cited as basic in the same sense as hunger, sleep, and sex needs. (The need for isolation, though feared, is a pathologic deviation occurring in schizoids and schizophrenics.) If a comparatively normal (although neurotic!) personality is forced into isolation, a feeling of loneliness ensues.

Death, being of course the ultimate separation, may be seen by the individual as an enforced total isolation, an experience in which he must go out of this world unaccompanied, unloved, not missed (an extension of the hated life situation)—completely and irrevocably alone. This may tend considerably to enhance the original basic fear of death. The individual, still healthily alive, multiplies his anxieties in the face of the ultimate loneliness of death.

Anger

Death to some means loss of substance, loss of that which they have spent a lifetime painstakingly building. Death destroys their labors by destroying and dissolving their substance (concretely, the body; abstractly, the soul). The reactive feeling is anger. The child who builds a house of blocks, and delights in the growing structure, is an apt illustration. He becomes aware of his creativity, and he is absorbed by it. Along comes someone who carelessly or unthinkingly pushes against it and causes the house to fall. With what dismay and what anger does the child react to this shocking destruction! In the same sense let us think of the adult who builds, in material and spiritual terms, the structure of his personality. Along comes Death and knocks over his construction, his substance, as though it were indeed a house of blocks. Here the "builder" is an adult, not a child. His rational adult mind does not permit him to recognize the anger against that force which may at any moment dissolve his structure through death. Since anger or fury toward death seems too irrational to countenance, it is transformed into a generally accepted, rationally understandable feeling: Fear.

The reverse may also happen. Fear may be so intolerable as to be transformed into a substitutive reaction: Anger. A forty-two-year-old patient was aptly nicknamed "The Angry Angel." He believed himself to be basically a very kind person, and was distressed by chronic anger reactions which he could not understand. Here again a dream revealed the origin of what proved to be the cause of his anger. It had occurred with some regularity since the patient was nine years old.

A ghostly, oversized machine, almost human, rolls toward me. I want

to escape, but find no hiding place. I try to resist the machine but it
is a futile struggle, and soon I am paralyzed. I recover and go into a
rage, but in vain. I end up with a terrific fear which I cannot throw off.

At the age of nine, the patient had seen his dead aunt in her
coffin. ("This sight was the fright of my life. That night I had the
dream for the first time.") We see here the sterile endeavor of this
person, as boy and as man, to resist the death idea. Fury became
the concomitant of his fear. He could not rid himself of either
until, in therapy, he discovered the connection.

Death as an Enemy

A painting by Dürer portrays Death as a strangler—his victim is
being throttled. This dramatic representation of death as an enemy
has a parallel in the secret fears of people who fear death as a
human enemy is hated and feared. This paranoid demonstration
(Death is an enemy who will try to harm me) is found mainly in
persons suspicious of others. They attempt to suppress their own
homicidal tendencies by projecting them onto others, and ultimately onto the final enemy, Death. Paradoxically, death is here in
some sense personified because there is at work at the same time
the need to depersonify the human enemy. The factor of the
human enemy is thus set aside, and life with other human beings
thereby made a little more tenable.

Possessiveness

Those people whose strong characteristic is possessiveness are especially disturbed by the fear of death. They cannot let go in life,
and they cannot let go *of* life. Letting go, to these people, represents defeat. Thus, letting go of life means to be defeated by the
conqueror, death—and defeat is what they are least able to accept.
The fear of death becomes unconsciously equated with the fear of
defeat.

Denial of Fear of Death

This writer, having become very conscious in her therapeutic
practice of the role which the fear of death plays in the neurotic

personality, could not believe a particular patient who claimed to have no such fear. The patient, a woman of fifty with phobic reactions, tenaciously denied ever in her life having experienced any fear of physical death. She was undoubtedly convinced of the truth of her own statement.

> Her first recollection dated back to the age of five. In the remembered incident, the child, upon the departure of her mother for a short trip, had crept forlornly under the piano. In this hiding place she had wept and implored her absent mother, "Mother, come home! The angel is trying to get me!" Her fear of being carried away by the angel (undoubtedly Death) became so overwhelming that she could not live with it and had to push it out of the way. The fear was displaced and affixed to the movement of travel (flying, train-riding)—to the mother's trip, so to speak, as the cause, rather than to the fear of death which the absence of the protective parent had aroused. This displacement by the patient was a device by which she felt she safeguarded her sanity.

Insomnia

Death anxiety manifests itself physically in those prone to psychobiologic disturbances, one of which may be insomnia. Some insomniacs are afraid that death may catch them asleep, although they are unaware of this feeling on a conscious level. Sleep is a state in which the sleeper is not "at the controls." Anything, goes the unconscious rationale, can happen during this defenseless state, without one's own volition. Frequently these people have suffered severe feelings of intellectual inferiority since childhood. They feel that, in order to maintain what is at best a precarious control, they must remain awake.

Obesity

> An obese patient of thirty-one had, as a child, seen a dying neighbor whom she remembered as "a stout woman before she took sick." For the patient, the loss of weight which had so impressed her, became identical with dying. The slimness which she consciously desired was fraught with an unconscious significance of approaching death. She counteracted the hidden death fear by overeating to retain the stout appearance which she equated with health and life. As a result of her

insight, she reduced her weight considerably without going on a specific diet.

Fear of the Hereafter

There are those who seek solace from the distress of this life (and from the unacknowledged fear of death) by the thought of a Hereafter in which all will be good, and in which recompense will be made for the ills suffered in the mortal world. In this way they seek to comfort themselves in the face of present troubles, some even going so far as to find a rationale for a do-nothing attitude. What purpose is there in creativity or achievement if this life is but transitory, and the reward is after all going to come in the next?

But there are those who can find no comfort in thoughts of the Hereafter. It is an unknown quantity like death itself, and holds unimaginable terrors. In the mind of such a person the thought of the Hereafter becomes a two-edged sword. He wonders with Shakespeare's Hamlet:

> ... To die, to sleep;
> To sleep: perchance to dream: aye, there's the rub;
> For in that sleep of death what dreams may come,
> When we have shuffled off this mortal coil,
> Must give us pause ...

In this connection, my own personal experience may be of some interest. Before undergoing major surgery, I had asked my nurse's cooperation in recording any dreams that I might have and report them to me after the operation. The following dream was recorded:

> I see myself watching my own funeral. The road to the cemetery is uphill. The cemetery is invisible because of the hill, but I know that the grave awaits me there. Many people are walking uphill in the funeral procession. I recognize a few of them. I hear the bells tolling and am pleased by the sonorous sounds as I have always been on hearing them. I think to myself, "These are the bells of Peace!" My only worry is the thought that pain, emotional and physical, might be in store for me after death. I appeal to the people attending my funeral, especially those whom I recognize, "Please help me. I don't mind dying, but I am concerned that I may have pain afterward. It isn't fair to let a person suffer after death. I don't know what you can do, but please take care of me and don't let me suffer after death."

I had always supposed my own concept of death to be one of complete dissolution and nothingness. This dream, which was so utterly contrary to my belief, came therefore as a complete surprise. It indicated strongly that preoccupation with thoughts of the Hereafter may exist on a subterranean level, in complete opposition to that which ar individual believes his own concept to be.

Summary

This paper has been concerned primarily with the obligation of the psychotherapist to take cognizance of the universality, whether conscious or repressed, of anxiety regarding death. The writer has provided, from her own therapeutic work with patients, some examples of the guises under which the fear of death may be hidden.

Death is variously viewed as a complete loss of power, a defeat, a deprivation of free will which destroys the creative capacity. It is goal-less and static; it represents non-being, nothingness. It means psychobiologic separation and isolation. It annihilates the godlike self-image of ominiscience, omnipotence, omnipresence, and immortality. It is the attack of a satanic enemy, a verdict pronounced at any moment without process. It provides no alternative other than to end life's death-wait by means of suicide.

There are as many defenses against the fear of death as there are conceptualizations. Some people dwarf the issue; some repress it; some desensitize themselves in order not to feel the pangs. Some allow the fear of or hopelessness about death to overshadow their lives. Some avoid naming it (taboo). Some fear the prospect of eternal silence. Some are consoled by a belief in the Hereafter, while for others the same belief conjures up nameless terrors. Some, such as scientists, believe in perfect dissolution, a state of non-being which embraces only nothingness, while to others such a state is inconceivable yet terrifying. Some refuse to think about death at all; others think of death before all else.

All of these notions deserve intensive analytic investigation. The discussion of the patient's own conceptualization of death must necessarily be an integral part of the psychotherapeutic procedure. The conference of therapist and patient serves to elucidate feelings, open or hidden, that surround the concept of death and are usually linked with other significant feelings, unnecessarily fortifying the basic death anxiety.

Negative character traits activate the fear and attendant anxieties and produce phobic reaction formations. Psychophysical ills are frequently based on disguised fears of death. They are amenable to cure if properly and profoundly dealt with in therapy.

As the personality develops toward maturity as a total entity, less and less is it overshadowed by the prospect of death. If a high degree of integration can be achieved, the prognosis for reducing neurotic fears of death to a normal level is excellent.

REFERENCES

1. MAY, R. "Contributions of Existential Psychotherapy." In *Existence, a New Dimension in Psychiatry and Psychology,* May, R., Angel, E., and Ellenberger, H. F., Eds. New York: Basic Books, 1958.
2. ADLER, A. *The Individual Psychology of Alfred Adler,* Ansbacher, H. L., and Ansbacher, R. R., Eds. New York: Basic Books, 1956.
3. HORNEY, K. *New Ways in Psychoanalysis.* New York: W. W. Norton, 1953.
4. GREENBERG, I. M. and ALEXANDER, I. E. "Some Correlates of Thoughts and Feelings Concerning Death." *J. Hillside Hosp.,* 11 (1962), p. 120.
5. ROSENTHAL, H. "Psychotherapy for the Dying." *Am. J. Psychother.,* 11 (1957): 616.
6. KINGMAN, R. "Fears and Phobias," Part II. *Welfare,* 19 (1928), p. 303.
7. ZILBOORG, G. "Fear of Death." *Psychoanalyt. Quart.,* 12 (1943), p. 465.
8. GORDON, R. "The Death Instinct and Its Relation to the Self." *J. Analyt. Psychol.,* 6 (1961), p. 119.
9. WAHL, C. W. "The Fear of Death." *Bull. Menninger Clin.,* 22 (1958), p. 214.
10. ARONSON, M. L., FURST, H. B., *et. al.* "The Impact of the Death of a Leader on a Group Process." *Am. J. Psychother.,* 16 (1962), p. 460.
11. FREUD, S. "Beyond the Pleasure Principle." In *The Standard Edition of the Complete Psychological Works of Sigmund Freud,* Vol. 18. Strachey, J., Ed. London: Hogarth Press, 1955.
12. WILLIAMS, M. "The Fear of Death," Part II. *J. Analyt. Psychol.,* 7 (1962), p. 29.
13. EISSLER, K. R. *The Psychiatrist and the Dying Patient.* New York: International Universities Press, 1955.
14. HOWARD, J. D. "Fear of Death." *J. Indiana State Med. Ass.,* 54 (1961), p. 1773.
15. ADLER, A. *The Practice and Theory of Individual Psychology.* New York & London: Humanities Press, 1951.
16. FROMM-REICHMANN, F. "Psychiatric Aspects of Anxiety." In *Psychoanalysis and Psychotherapy,* Bullard, D. M., Ed. Chicago: University of Chicago Press, 1959.

MOURNING

I. EROS AND
THE TRAUMA OF DEATH

HARRY SLOCHOWER

In *The Psychiatrist and The Dying Patient* (1)—a perceptive study which has yet to receive proper evaluation—K. R. Eissler notes that man is the only species which knows death, and that this knowledge shapes his life. Possibly, it shapes his life even more than the oedipus complex.

Preoccupation with death has a unique character in our time. Death is a major theme in modern philosophy from Schopenhauer and Nietzsche to Heidegger and Sartre. It is a focus for many modern and contemporary writers and artists from Novalis to Thomas Mann and the theatre of "the absurd." We see it in painting from the expressionists (especially Karl Hofer) and Pablo Picasso. And, since Freud's publication of *Beyond the Pleasure Principle* (1920), the subject has been receiving increasing attention in psychology, notably George B. Wilbur, Norman O. Brown, Paul Friedman, Joost Meerloo, Herman Feifel and K. R. Eissler.

Freud holds that the unconscious harbors no image of our own death. It would follow that the death drive is not "inborn," that no one wants to die. The idea that, "by nature," we all want to live is put forth in Spinoza's famous principle of "conatus."

In his *Ethics* (III, Prop. VII), Spinoza states: "Everything, insofar as it is in itself, endeavors to persist in its own being."

Yet, just as the question of "to be" is decided for us when we are born, so the question of "not to be" is answered by our past history in which all that was born, died. To counter this melancholy fate, man has made manifold attempts to "circumvent" death or to find some consolations for it—by religion, philosophy, mysticism, art and psychology.

Historical Consolations

Jacques Choron's recent study *Death and Western Philosophy* (2) presents a lucid and informed account of philosophical attitudes toward death, from antiquity to the contemporary era. The account discloses the various strategies used to find consolations or compensations for death.

Primitive man attempted to circumvent death by identifying himself with his clan and tribe. There was a shared belief that where a person felt himself part of his collective community, he "lived" before he was born and "lived on" after his individual decease. Ernst Cassirer quotes the anthropologist Elsdon Best, who reports a primitive as saying: "I defeated the enemy"—referring to his tribe which had defeated an enemy hundreds of years ago.

With the development of individuation, manifested in the rise of mythopoesis, we meet a "revolt" against death. In the Babylonian epic of Gilgamesh, the hero refuses to accept the death of his friend Enkidu, then journeys himself in a quest for the plant of immortality. Egyptian literature and art attempt to deny death. Breasted notes that the word "death" does not occur in the Pyramid texts, except when referring to the enemy. And Egyptian embalmings, tombs, pyramids and embellishments of the dead were intended as physical "proofs" that the dead had not died.

Greek art pictured death as the brother of sleep. In Plato's dialogues, Socrates maintains serenity when confronted by his death sentence. He states in the *Phaedo* that "the real philosopher has reason to be of good cheer when he is about to die . . ." for the soul is immortal. He concludes that "those who pursue philosophy rightly study to die." The Middle Ages developed this point on a theological plane, finding solace in the belief that the soul lives on after death, and that even the sinner can be saved by sufficient or efficient grace. Schopenhauer's metaphysics offered a pantheistic consolation which transposed the primitive identification with the tribe to the individual's merging with the cosmic Will. And, since such identification was, for Schopenhauer, the highest goal, he called death "the true inspiring genius, or the muse of philosophy." Mann's Thomas Buddenbrook is one of the last characters in literature who seeks—vainly—such Schopenhauerian consolation.

Contemporary Idolatries: Gadgetry and Doctor Strangelove

The universality of the life-death drive, like any other general concept, must always be examined in *statu nascendi*. Applying this principle, we need to ask what specific forces in our present scene tend to intensify or reduce these drives. We know that Freud's own theory of the death instinct was developed under the impact of the First World War.

In an essay, *War Within Man* (3), Erich Fromm gives an eloquent statement of the thesis that today people "are not afraid of total destruction because they do not love life." Pleasure and excitement are the advertised ultimate objectives; but they are without living substance. In the nineteenth century, Marx had argued that industrial capitalism gives primacy to the fetishism of commodities and Emerson complained then that "things ride mankind." In our century, Franz Kafka, writing in an era of developing "automation," symbolized and allegorized the *human* inefficiency of mechanical "efficiency."

Kafka wrote before automation developed unmanned missiles, before the appearance of the atomic, hydrogen and neutron bomb. The bomb introduces a new Moloch of archaic nature, unpredictable, perhaps unknowable and uncontrollable. This power makes a Nirvana of universal death a near certainty. Individual or even collective responsibility for such a cosmic Armaggedon is reduced to insignificance: It needs but one finger pressing a button thousands of miles away.

The incalculable power and pervasive presence of the machine has not only caught men up in a mechanical reflex action, including its "pleasures" (as seen, for example, in the routinized sex motions in the Beatnik and other contemporary fiction). It has also brought a strange identification with and fascination for this mechanical monster.

This is the terrifying theme in the movie version of James Jones' *The Thin Red Line* and, more perceptively, in the film *Doctor Strangelove* [written by Stanley Kubrick, Terry Southern and Peter George, based on the novel *Red Alert* by Peter George]. What we have here is the nightmarish picture of a doctor who falls in "love" with the godlike omnipotence of the lethal bomb, the secular church of scientism. In Eugene O'Neill's *Dynamo*,

Reuben Light leaves his Protestant religious home to discover the new God, electricity. Yet, even as the new deity is the product of man's reason and the nature of science is to give precise and unambiguous answers, the dynamo refuses to communicate with man. Its power alone communicates. Where O'Neill's character is disappointed in being left solely with facing the mystery of electric power, Doctor Strangelove is seized by a delirious enthusiasm for the even more enigmatic and more pervasive power of the bomb.

The picture of the people around Doctor Strangelove is terrifying on another level. Where the doctor identifies with the excitement of worldwide catastrophe and *Menschendämmerung,* the others have identified with the mechanistic rhythm to the point where they themselves react in this rhythm, so that no one feels able or is willing to try and counter the impending doom. One gets the feeling that no human hand or heart can stop this impersonal Moloch or Golem. Death may come at any instant, no human being is responsible or guilty. The resultant feeling is one of apathy and indifference for "the decision" is out of human hands. It fills one with absence of communication, with absence of a meaningful future, with life as death. Even the *living* element of thanatophobia tends to be dulled. Such indifference, apathy, impotence and shifting of responsibility was manifested in the incident in which some two dozen New York residents failed to make as much as a telephone call in response to a young woman's screams that she was being stabbed. It crops up in some forms of juvenile delinquency. See my paper "The Juvenile Delinquent and the Mythic Hero" (*Dissent,* Summer 1961).

The Narcissistic Eros, Time and Thanatos

Legend has it that Narcissus brought destruction not only to himself, but also to others and to both men and women. For his destructive self-absorption, Narcissus was made to fall in love, but was denied fulfillment of his love. Narcissus' uncontrolled sexual passion has affinity to Eros. The son of the sister-brother deities, Zeus and Aphrodite, Eros exemplifies the recurrent mythic motifs of incest.

In a major article on Freud's life-death instinct, George B. Wilbur makes the point that "the death instinct is a necessary consequence of the life instinct, Eros," that the concept is presumably a consequence of "the concept of narcissism," adding that the ancient myth offers here additional support (4).

The feeling of helplessness and apparent apathy has its polar counterpart: an explosive dynamism, itself born of and expressing this same helplessness. [Possibly, those who shout, "Jump! Jump!" when they watch someone perched to jump from a roof, etc., are motivated by a desire to have someone perform *an act of decision,* having the character of finality.] It was foreshadowed by the "transition" movement ("time is a tyranny to be abolished") and by the Futurists with their apotheosis of "frenzy," of "aggressive movement . . . to increase the enthusiastic fervor of the primordial elements."

Current preoccupation with Thanatos is tied to obsession with Eros. This Eros is under the aegis of a narcissistic "pleasure principle," set to a furious, restless "rock and roll" pace—the contemporary version of the Bacchantes. This tendency to live in a *Rausch,* to "live it up" alternates with and results in a "living it down." The "pleasure principle" harbors within itself "the beyond—" of the pleasure principle. The contemporary Eros merges into Thanatos dress or, one could say, that the Thanatos drive assumes the form of a frenzied narcissistic Eros.

This Eros is bound up with the ritual of time and money ("time is money"). It would "buy" everything, life and love. And, it would buy time, the 24 hours or years ever sold by the evil one from Marlowe's Mephistopheles to Mann's devil in *Doctor Faustus.* In *Wilhelm Meister,* Goethe called time "a gift of God," and in a Dionysian temper, he celebrated the living process as a flaming death *(Flammentod):*

> Das Lebendige will ich preisen,
> Das nach Flammentod sich sehnet.

At the close of his life, when Goethe was concluding his *Faust,* and under the impact of developing industrial capitalism, time becomes an ambiguous gift. As he is about to die ("Die Uhr steht still"), Faust is told by Sorge that all his life, he had been blind to the fact that his homage to time and restless striving made for his perpetual unease. At this point, she blinds Faust. (Vision was symbolic for highest life values to Goethe. Legend has it that his last words were: "Mehr Licht!").

Nietzsche underwent a similar development. His Superman champions never-ceasing willing and surpassing. In his later phase, Nietzsche tired of this pace and, in a poem, he questions it, asking himself: "Lief ich zu rasch meines Weges . . .?" Nietzsche then proceeded to "correct" this linear temper by the doctrine of a circular Eternal Recurrence. Psychologically, this is a form of repetion compulsion and the other pole of temporal progress. Similarly, in Thomas Mann's *Magic Mountain,* Settembrini's homage to time and progress merges with Naphta's homage to eternity and death, and in *Doctor Faustus,* Mann's Andreas Leverkuhn "buys time" at the price of ending in regressed timelessness.

Freud: To Die "Nur Auf Seine Weise."

In "Instincts and their Vicissitudes" (5), Freud indicated a connection between hate and love and held that hate was older than love.

The question of which came "first"—Eros or Thanatos—is an undialectic posing of the problem and is, in this sense, uncharacteristic of the Freudian methodology. If Life and Love are to be examined in their full "implications," they point to their negative, their opposite and contrary. In his more representative formulation, Freud presented the concatenation of life and death. His admonition: "Si vis vitam, para mortem" ("If one wishes life, one should prepare for death"), expresses their interconnection in epigrammatic form. (Joan Riviere's translation in *Collected Papers,* Vol. 4, p. 317 is: "If you would endure life, be prepared for death.")

In *Beyond the Pleasure Principle,* Freud wrote that the goal of life is discovered in death. This statement is generally interpreted as meaning that one of man's basic urges is to die. Yet, even as Freud maintained that man's tendency is to return to his ancient starting point, he introduced two crucial modifications: First, that "everything living dies for *internal* reasons" (p.V.—my emphasis). Second, that the organism wishes to die "in its own fashion" ("nur auf seine Weise" [6]—To die in its own fashion). These points (as Gotthardt Booth, Laci Fessler and R. R. Eissler have recognized) mean: Man wants to choose *how* he is to die. He does not wish a death decided from without and by others. [In *Ego and the Id,*

ch. IV, Freud notes: "We perceive that for the purposes of discharge the instinct of destruction is habitually brought into the
service of Eros."] Man is "ready" for death when he has fulfilled
and expressed the powers of his being, has reached the point when
he can no longer incorporate new experiences, that is, can no
longer *grow*. He is then "free" to die. This thought has affinity to
the concept of freedom as conceptualized by Spinoza and Hegel.

Eissler's book *The Psychiatrist and the Dying Patient* presents
case histories of two patients each of whom knew that their can-
cerous disease was fatal and who had no recourse to religious,
philosophical or mystic consolations. The study raises the difficult
and delicate task of how the analyst can help such patients. We
speak of "fear" about death. Yet, properly viewed, we are dealing
not with fear, but with a desire to live *out* one's existence to its
fullest dimensions. The problem is not fear of death, but of
wanting to live on in a dignified and human fashion.

Toward the end, Shakespeare's Hamlet speaks the line: "The
readiness is all" (In *King Lear* he says, "Ripeness is all"). Hamlet
here expresses his readiness for death. But his tone is melancholy
for Hamlet had not been able to develop a readiness for choosing
an integrated life. His "readiness" is not the result of irreducible
human tragedy, is not *la condition humaine,* such as we meet in
classical tragedy and mythopoesis.

Dante and Rilke

Freud acknowledged that poets have anticipated some of the
basic insights of psychoanalysis. On the problem of life and death,
Dante and Rilke represent startling instances.

Dante's *Divine Comedy* would have it that human fate after
death is determined by the way man has lived. However, the real
relevance is to life on earth. For what Dante calls the "practical"
import of his epic is this: Earlier actions set the pattern for later
behavior. Hence Dante urges: "Think of the sequel."

The work of Rainer Maria Rilke reveals some startling parallels
to Freudian concepts.

In his comprehensive and psychoanalytically penetrating study
of Rilke (7), Erich Simenauer offers evidence that Rilke had a
knowledge of Freud's theories, but that his attitude toward analysis

was ambivalent. Rilke was afraid of psychoanalysis for a reason, similar to Kafka's. Both felt that a clarification of the unconscious motives and process of their work would lame their impulse to produce. Rilke writes: "Put in a somewhat exaggerated form, my feeling is this: I would have to stop working as soon as anyone were able to clarify my *relation to my work,* its nature, *its source,* its process." (Letter of Oct. 4, 1907; cited by Simenauer, p. 117). Simenauer would show that Rilke had a strong tendency toward a "feminine masochism," especially evident in *The Notebooks of Malte Laurids Brigge.* However—and this needs to be stressed—such genetic data do not explain the vibrant and incantatory qualities of Rilke's poetry. (These are stressed in Walther Rehm's *Orpheus* [8]. Here, however, Rilke's personality profile dissolves into a nebulous mythic symbolism.)

Rilke's poetry is a lyric rendition of the polarity of the life-death process. Aside from the Third Book of *Das Stunden-Buch,* two volumes of poetry are devoted to the subject of death: *Sonnets to Orpheus* and *Duineser Elegien* (the latter followed Rilke's journey to Egypt in 1913 and gives an appreciation of the Egyptian cult of the dead). Rilke evokes the imagery of the moon to represent the fullness and circularity of existence—containing both the side which we see and the side which is turned away from us. Rilke, too, saw that death was deeply imbedded in the nature of love and writes that if one loves life generously enough, then one draws into oneself life's other half, death. In the 13th sonnet of the Second Part of the Orpheus Sonnets, we read that being is the condition for non-being:

> Sei—und wisse zugleich des Nicht-Seins Bedingung . . .

Rilke's *Stunden-Buch* distinguishes between a death which is "authentic" and one (as in the big cities) which is "small":

> Dort ist der Tod . . .
> der kleine Tod . . .
> wie eine Frucht in ihnen, die nicht reift.*

In the *Notebooks of Malte Laurids Brigge,* Rilke bewails the fact today "the wish to have a death of one's own is growing ever

*There is death . . .
Small death . . .
In them, a fruit that does not ripen.

rarer." This is what makes dying alien and difficult: "that it is not our death":

> Denn dieses macht das Sterben fremd und schwer,
> dass es nicht *unser* Tod ist; einer der
> uns endlich nimmt, weil wir keinen reifen.†

And Rilke's monk pleads with the Lord that he give each person "his own death," a death which is an expression and development from within and issues from a life which knew love, meaning and suffering:

> O Herr, gib jedem seinen eignen Tod,
> Das Sterben, das aus jenem Leben geht,
> darin er Liebe hatte, Sinn und Not . . .‡

Such death is likened to ripeness:

> . . . Sie wollten blühn,
> Und blühn ist schön sein; doch wir wollen reifen . . .**

> [*Das Stunden-Buch*]

Similarly, Nietzsche had written that all which is ripe wants to die and that the important thing was to die at the right time. Time—the category of "progress" without final standards—was Rilke's "deepest woe" ("Die Zeit ist mir mein tiefstes Weh . . ."). The dead are "souls in space." Rilke's work is an attempt to rescue space from being devoured by time, prevent permanence from being splintered into successiveness.

Philosophic-Mythic Dialectic

The dialectic operative in the life-death rhythm has long been recognized by philosophers since Heracleitus. We find it in Hegel

†For this makes dying strange and difficult,
   That it is not *our* death; a death
   That takes us in the end, because we reach no ripeness.

‡O Lord, give to each man his own death,
   That death that grows out of that living,
   Wherein he loved and grew to wisdom, suffered.

**. . . They seek to bloom;
   To bloom is to be lovely; still, we desire our ripeness . . .

Translated by E. Louise Mally

and, in our own day, in Max Scheler and Martin Heidegger. Scheler saw death as part of the organic process in life itself. For Heidegger, "being-in-the-world" constitutes being "thrown into death," is *Sein zum Tode*. To understand Being, one must begin with death. Both "anxiety" *(Angst)* and death are necessary corollaries of "being-in-the-world as such." (Heidegger, like Freud before him, distinguishes between fear and anxiety, but sees anxiety as an "existential" or ontic problem, rather than as a psychological issue.) And, in his notion of "freedom-toward-death," Heidegger suggests that by recognizing that death is part of life, man can incorporate death and thereby free himself from its full terror and for "resoluteness."

In *The Science of Logic* (I, 142), Hegel states that the hour of birth is the hour of death. Only finite things experience birth, and to be born means to be finite. Another way of putting it: "To be" means to be limited, incomplete, imperfect. Only non-being is unlimited, complete, finished and perfect. This point is suggested by the Hebrew *tam,* which is related to the antithetical word *mas.* The first means "perfect"; the second means "death." In Thomas Mann's *Joseph the Provider,* Joseph is *tam,* and this signifies (Mann writes) that he is both "light and dark, life and death . . . the upper and the under world at once and by turns." Indeed, the word "per-fection" points to death, the word connoting an act "finished."

In clinical practice, we meet with mourning and "death"-feelings on the parts of patients. This transpires, at times, prior to their readiness for transformation of their personality in which they incorporate their "death" in a new type of life. Such, for example, is the experience of Goethe's Faust as he descends to the depths of "the Mothers." Such is the desperate hope of Mann's Andreas Leverkuhn, who lives through the Nazi terror. Such transfiguration is a recurrent motif in the ritual of the seasonal god of mythopoesis, with its notion that death is part of the rhythm of birth and rebirth. [Even as Erich Fromm has written perceptively on certain aspects of mythic motifs, his tendency to draw sharp diremptions between "normal biology" and pathology leads him to regard a return "to the darkness of the womb" and the death instinct as wholly negative.]

The example of Mann's Leverkuhn illuminates the uniqueness

of the problem of death in an age of Fascism, followed by the hellish bomb. The new archaic juggernaut cannot be met solely by philosophical or religious consolation. Nor is psychological analysis of the individual enough. These must be joined with group analysis and with collective, organized activity. In this way, the issues raised by death which Eissler calls "possibly the foremost problem of the mind," can be approached functionally. For, the "pity of it" is that today *tragic* death is nearly impossible. When death comes through chance, absurdity, maniacal acting out or an impersonal "enemy," there is only pity.

These intractable exigencies of history impose a trivial and tenuous character on the problem of death. To be sure, history also offers the opportunity for a death which has a kind of lapidary dignity. There is dignity in a death which comes as a consequence of fighting for social and individual freedom or for the life and liberty of one's beloved (9). Such dignity was exemplified, during the days of the Nazi wrath, by those who fought and died in the Warsaw ghetto, at Stalingrad, on the beaches of Normandy, and in the liberation of Paris.

Yet, beyond temporal pressures, man perennially faces the ineluctable certainty that "all men are mortal." Whereas we become aware of death very early, some never gain awareness of oedipal involvements. The oedipal problem is subject to degrees of resolution. It can be attenuated and "lived" with. Some can go "beyond the oedipus complex." But, there is no resolution, attenuation or "living" with death. And one cannot go "beyond" it, for it is itself the beyond. With time, its spectral shadow spreads and, no matter how well "analyzed," hangs in some measure over the life of every man. Every time we confront it in fact or in knowledge, we undergo a measure of traumatic experience. The "trauma of birth" occurs only once. The trauma of death is experienced over and over again in the course of a man's lifetime. The *knowledge* of death is the most continuous, most persistent and inevitable, perhaps the most fateful trauma for man.

REFERENCES

1. K. R. EISSLER. *The Psychiatrist and the Dying Patient*. New York: International Universities Press, 1955.
2. JACQUES CHORON. *Death and Western Philosophy*. New York: Collier Books, 1963.
3. ERICH FROMM. *War Within Man*. American Friends Service Committee, 1963 (Pamphlet).
4. GEORGE B. WILBUR. "Some Problems Presented By Freud's Life-Death Instinct Theory." *American Imago*, Vol. II, No. 3, pp. 251ff.
5. S. FREUD. *Collected Papers*, 4, 76f., 82. ("Instincts and Their Vicissitudes").
6. S. FREUD. *Gesammelte Werke*, London: Imago Publ. Co., 1940, Vol. XIII, p. 14.
7. ERICH SIMENAUER. *Rainer Maria Rilke. Legende und Mythos*. Frankfurt am Main: Schauinsland-Verlag, 1953.
8. WALTHER REHM. *Orpheus. Der Dichter und die Toten*. Dusseldorf: Verlag L. Schwann, 1950, pp. 379–671.
9. For other forms or "deflections" that the idea of death reveals as a literary theme, see Kenneth Burke's essay "Thanatopsis for Critics" in *Essays in Criticism*, October 1952.
10. HARRY SLOCHOWER. *Literature and Philosophy Between Two World Wars (No Voice Is Wholly Lost)*. New York: Citadel Press, 1964 (Paperback).

II. THE SORROW
OF BEREAVEMENT

HOWARD BECKER

A great deal of attention has been paid by ethnographers to the intense fear of death and the dead manifested by "savages." It may be, however, that preliterates mourn for the deceased in quite as loving and sorrowful a fashion as we do, but that the early observers, many of whom were missionaries with well-defined standards of propriety for all the great crises of life, recorded only the "heathenish" and "outlandish" aspects of mourning cere-monies and funeral rites. Be that as it may, the fact remains that most of the accounts we have stress the presence of the fear element in mourning and disposal customs, so that any discussion of what Shand calls the "laws of sorrow"[1] must focus upon the literate peoples who have left their own records—who have not had to trust to the tender mercies of the more or less unsympathetic observer.

Because of these written records, we have a rich store of materials at hand for the analysis of the social psychology of bereavement among literate groups. Although these materials are not organized in so-called scientific or academic form, they are none the less valuable. McDougall says on this point: "I shall use the term 'psychology' and 'psychologist' to denote the scientific varieties; but in doing so, I shall imply no disrespect for the achievements in this sphere of poets and biographers and writers of romance. The wise psychologist will regard literature as a vast storehouse of information about human experience, and will not neglect to draw from it what he can."[2]

The psychologist who up to date has made what many scholars regard as the most effective use of the vast store of material, ancient and modern, which illustrates the workings of the primary emotion of sorrow is A. E. Shand, in his book *The Foundations of Char-*

acter. Shand differs from McDougall in his classification of the primary tendencies and emotions, although fundamentally they begin at the same point. He has, as primary emotions, fear, anger, disgust, wonder, joy, and sorrow; and as the goal-seeking tendencies (instincts) connected with each of these emotions respectively he has flight and concealment, combat or pugnacity, repulsion, the maintenance of a pleasurable process already existing, curiosity, and aversion or repugnance. He classes hunger and sex as appetites, not as goal-seeking tendencies, and introduces another category which he calls impulses, needs, or wants, and in which he places exercise and repose.

Any or all of these emotions, tendencies, appetites, or impulses may be organized in the greater systems of the sentiments. For example, according to Shand, parental love, a sentiment, includes in its system nutritive, defensive, sportive, and offensive "instincts," using the latter term to cover appetites, impulses, and goal-seeking tendencies or instincts proper. The same sentiment may include in its organization, at one time or another, all of the important primary emotions of fear, anger, joy, and sorrow.

This brief indication of the general nature of Shand's theory will suffice for our purposes here. The fact significant for the present study is that whatever the outcome of the instinct-controversy may be, Shand, by the use of these thought forms, has arrived at certain empirical principles which can be used as categories for grouping various extremely complex forms of behavior. He calls them (rather grandiloquently, to be sure), "laws," but claims nothing more for them than this: "How long it took me before I saw the necessity of being content with good working hypotheses! Hence, as I only try to find such hypotheses, to interpret the facts of character as far as I have grasped them, I do not put them forward in the form of finally adequate theories. . . . And I have sought to give them such form that they can be made use of by others without being wholly abandoned."[3]

About a fifth of Shand's book is given over to a discussion of sorrow, and it is to this that our attention will be directed. The balance of this article will be devoted to a greatly condensed exposition of the theories and empirical principles therein contained, with illustrations drawn from case studies made by the writer (ten in all) and from a wide range of literary sources. The writer will

also offer a good deal of interpretation of the principles themselves. Of course, only such principles and illustrations of sorrow
as have a bearing on the social psychology of bereavement will be
considered.[4]

Sorrow is extremely difficult to interpret and analyze; its variety
of expression is perhaps greater than that of any other primary
emotion, so that sometimes there seems to be a real difference in
kind between its diverse manifestations.

There is, for instance, the sorrow that gives free vent to its
violence in outward behavior. In this sort we have a close resemblance to some preliterate "frenzied" mourning customs, where
widows scarify their faces or brothers beat each other over the
head with jagged clubs. One example among many must suffice:

> She willfully her sorrow did augment
> And offered hope of comfort did despise;
> Her golden locks most cruelly she rent,
> And scratched her face with ghastly dreriment;
> Ne would she speak, ne yet be seene,
> But hid her visage, and her head down bent.[5]

Then, besides the violent kind, there is the sort that is tearless
and mute. DeQuincey in interpreting this says: "The sentiment
which attends the sudden revelation that all is lost! silently is
gathered up into the heart; it is too deep for gestures or for words;
and no part of it passes to the outside."[6] Some illustrations of this
type follow:

> I tell you, hopeless grief is passionless;
> That only men incredulous of despair,
> Half-taught in anguish, through the midnight air
> Beat upward in God's throne in loud access
> Of weeping and reproach. Full desertness
> In souls as countries lieth silent-bare
> Under the blanching, vertical eye-glare
> Of the absolute Heavens. Deep-hearted man, express
> Grief for thy Dead in silence like to death,
> Most like a monumental statue set
> In everlasting watch and moveless woe
> Till itself crumble to the dust beneath.
> Touch it; the marble eyelids are not wet;
> If it could weep, it would arise and go.[7]

My lighter moods are like to these
That out of words a comfort win;
But there are other griefs within,
And tears that at their fountain freeze.[8]

Home they brought her warrior dead;
She nor swoon'd nor utter'd cry.
All her maidens, watching, said,
She must weep, or she will die.[9]

O hearts that break and give no sign
Save whitening lip and fading tresses.[10]

Some of life's sad ones are too strong to die,
Grief doesn't kill them as it kills the weak,
Sorrow is not for those who sit and cry
Lapped in the love of turning t'other cheek,
But for the noble souls austere and bleak,
Who have had the bitter dose and drained the cup,
And wait for death face fronted, standing up.[11]

There is a third type of sorrow which is without either the impulsiveness of the first or the concentration and self-control of the second, but which sinks under the sense of weakness and discouragement. This is the sorrow which the physiologists describe as having a "paralysing action . . . over the voluntary muscles," and as accompanied by a "feeling of fatigue, or heaviness."[12] This type, while it is sometimes the immediate effect of misfortune, is also the subdued state into which violent sorrows pass after they have exhausted the individual. Some excerpts from case studies made by the writer illustrate this kind of sorrow with surprising aptness:

Most striking fact about after-effects of bereavement was lassitude of mind and body. Under strain for long time before suicide. When expected blow finally fell (she had made an attempt at taking her life about two years before, and continually talked about doing it again), felt as if load had been lifted, but no renewal of energy came—depression instead.

Necessity of attending to details of funeral, etc., seemed to enable husband to "carry on"; but after all was over, very marked slump in physical and mental energy. Formerly very methodical and neat, but just after funeral, and for some time, became "positively sloppy" in habits—nothing seemed to matter much; nothing not absolutely necessary evoked enough energy for carrying out. No appetite.

When body was finally interred there was marked "slump" in energy and ability to think—"everything was all over and nothing seemed of much use."

Felt in Epicurean frame of mind (not in popular sense) ; wanted to live unnoticed, as simply as possible. "Live and let live." Wanted no domestic responsibility—daughter an encumbrance. *General feebleness and self-indulgence.* Wanted to talk about situation to those who had not known wife. Compared feelings with another man who lost wife under tragic circumstances, and agreed on *numbing* effect of bereavement—seemed at times as though it had not been.

Again, a fourth type of sorrow frequently appears, the opposite of the third, for it is not accompanied by a feeling of fatigue or prostration, but by an activity approaching frenzy. This may seem somewhat like the first type, but in the first type the frenzy is directed against the individual himself; in the fourth it may be against others, as DeQuincey described it in the "Mater Tenebrarum."[13] Again, Lear curses his daughters in his grief, and cries, "O, let me not be mad, not mad, sweet heaven! Keep me in temper; I would not be mad."[14]

Varied as these four types are, however, they differ only in degree so far as the element of sorrow is concerned. Their contrasts are the result of temperament, extravert or introvert as the case may be, in differing measures. Habitual attitudes also may play a large part; the way in which the individual has obtained gratification of other thwarted desires may determine behavior when the wishes for response, etc., are thwarted by bereavement. Thus we may have the sullen type of sorrow, or the tantrum type, or even the combative type in which anger is directed upon an external "cause" or scapegoat, i.e., doctor, nurse, relatives, or God.

The first type, in which frenzy is directed against oneself, is perhaps less mixed with other sentiments than the others; the second is changed in outward form by the effect of self-control: our deepest love for others, as well as convention and the self-regarding sentiment, may lead us to restrain the expression of

emotions. The third type differs from the first chiefly by the
fatigue or prostration which marks it. Sorrow, when prolonged,
tends to have a depressing effect, even if, sometimes, its immediate
effect is stimulating.[15] The fourth is clearly a mixed type and
illustrates the frequent union of anger with sorrow in energetic
persons.

> The four types we have been considering are not then based on
> inherent differences of the tendencies or instincts comprised in
> sorrow . . . but merely on the different degrees of energy which belong
> to it, or on the degree in which it is controlled or elicits anger.[16]

Moreover, sadness, melancholy, Gray's "leuchocholy" and his
other sort, "black indeed,"[17] *Weltschmerz,* low spirits, melancholia,
and *melancholia agitans* (the latter two pathological) are all varieties of sorrow, but neither they nor the four varieties previously
considered disclose the essential nature of sorrow itself, because
all these manifestations can be shown to be determined either by
the influence of some extraneous system, such as anger or fear,
by fluctuations of the amount of energy present in the organism,
by basic temperamental trends, or by attitudinal habits. Consideration of these types therefore teaches us nothing concerning the
causation of sorrow—about its actual essence.

But our analysis has shown that when disconnected from other
influences *its varieties seem to be reducible to two, the depressed
and the excited,* and that these are conditioned by the degree of
the sorrow-producing stimulus on the one hand and the amount of
energy present to resist sorrow on the other—by the strength of
the *will-to-live,* which seeks the continuance of stimuli affording to
the organism a sense of the furtherance of life. Let us formulate
this conclusion as a principle of the causation of sorrow:

> (1) When either a primary impulse, or a desire, or a sentiment is
> frustrated, sorrow tends to be evoked, in proportion, other things
> equal, to the strength of the impulse, or desire, and the degree of its
> frustration.[18]

This is the first of the empirical principles which will be used in
this article. Assuming it to afford an adequate explanation of the
causation of sorrow, the next question is: What difference does
the occurrence of sorrow make to the impulse which has been
frustrated?

Shand answers this as follows:

> Sorrow appears to have one principal impulse—the cry for help or assistance. It is the emotion of weakness, the expression of failure. ... Sorrow is a system which possesses a characteristic impulse, first manifested in the infant's instinctive cry for help, a little later by watching its approaches; the cry itself becoming more distinctive of sorrow, and joining itself to articulate language, appealing for relief, distraction, sympathy.
>
> But yet we cannot rightly understand sorrow unless we bear in mind that though primary, and one of the first emotions, if not the first to be manifested in child-life, it is not independent, but is always related to a frustrated impulse, emotion, or sentiment which is the cause of its emotion; and that even where it wells up in us as a mood it must still imagine such frustration, in order to render its state intelligible.[19]

From this point on we shall cease following the analysis by which Shand arrives at his various empirical principles, and merely state the principles themselves with occasional comment.

> (2) The sorrow of love is ever attracted to the beloved object, and in diverse ways, strives to maintain all that remains of the former union.[20]

Literature is full of expressions of this universal tendency of sorrow at the loss of a loved object. When the attraction is opposed it becomes obstinate, and, like other obstructed impulses, often manifests anger. Rachel mourns for her children, and "will not be comforted." In the first stage of sorrow the attraction is so strong that bereaved persons may become "voluptuaries of grief," and may endeavor to maintain the painful remembrance of the object, and the painful state of sorrow itself. For example, a man who had lost a little boy says:

> Took walks with wife through parks and other places where child had played, and spoke to each other often—"Here's the place where Dick had such a good time that day," etc. This was too much of a strain—it was terrific. I coined a phrase to express the state we had drifted into; we were "voluptuaries of grief." We had no right to subject ourselves to that torture in the name of loyalty to the dead.[21]

> Mrs. Gummidge, in extenuation of her perpetual self-pity, says: "My troubles has made me contrary. I feel my troubles, and they make me contrary. I wish I didn't feel 'em, but I do. I wish I could be hardened

to 'em, but I can't . . ." Mr. Peggotty . . . looked round upon us, and
. . . said in a whisper: "She's been thinking of the old 'un!"[22]

And Tennyson, who calls sorrow "cruel fellowship," and "sweet
and bitter in a breath," yet invokes her to dwell with him, and be
"no casual mistress, but a wife."[23]

> Ah, sweeter to be drunk with loss,
> To dance with death, to beat the ground,
> Than that the victor hours should scorn
> The long result of love and boast,
> "Behold the man who loved and lost,
> But all he was is overworn."[24]

> Still onward winds the dreary way:
> I with it, for I long to prove
> No lapse of moons can canker love,
> Whatever fickle tongues may say.[25]

It must be noted that the type of sorrow so amply illustrated
is the "sorrow of love," and the next illustration tends to show
that where love is absent, there is no impulse of attraction to the
bereaved, nor is there any attempt to conserve memories. *Sorrow
there may be, but not the sorrow of love.*

This man, a case study of whom furnishes this example, had
lost all real love for his wife because she had erred sexually with
another man, and though he continued to live with her, and
retained somewhat of a "friendly feeling" toward her, real love
was absent. When her suicide finally occurred, his feelings took
the following form:

> When he first saw her dead body, there was no kissing or clinging to
> body—this might have happened if unfaithfulness had not taken
> "the bloom off the romance. She had always expressed desire for the
> more intangible and spiritual things in marriage, and then for the
> thing to happen that did happen—!" Memories of his wife, because
> of her unfaithfulness and the distressing circumstances of her death,
> were mostly unpleasant, and "I make a deliberate effort to bar
> them from my mind. The painful and interminable discussions of
> the last few months, and the psychopathic nature of her personality,
> with its intensity and strain and stress, make even my dreams of her
> very unpleasant." Wife made good deal of Christmas, so first Christ-
> mas after tragedy sent daughter to country and went away himself

to friend's in order to prevent memories. "When painful images came up, I willed not to think of them. It was a necessary means of self-defense." Glad to send clothing and other belongings to wife's people because of painful associations. Keeps things associated with her out of sight as much as possible. House took fire shortly after death; subject not altogether sorry this occurred, because it destroyed some mementoes would not otherwise have had courage to get rid of. Did not deliberately destroy anything, but would be glad "if some of the things wore out." Burned some of his letters to wife after suicide —after marriage had sometimes written every day when he or she was away—but cannot yet bring himself to burn her letters. Does not look at her pictures, which he keeps for form's sake, because spiritual break between them "too final, too irrevocable."[26]

So from these examples, both where love does and does not exist, it may certainly be restated that

"The sorrow of *love* is ever attracted to the beloved object, and in diverse ways, strives to maintain all that remains of the former union."

(3) The sorrow of love tends to restore that state of the beloved object, or that relation to it, the loss or destruction of which is the cause of the sorrow.[27]

And in the case of a man who lost his mother by death, we have a surprising variation of this same impulse of restoration:

Sight of upturned earth and grave evoked "a surprising reaction"— "most important thing I've got to tell you. When I was a little kid I was terribly afraid of death as soon as I got to know about it. I used to hope I'd be an exception to the general rule. Even in after life, I never got used to the idea, although I've cut up lots of 'stiffs.' But do you know, when I saw my mother tucked away down there in that grave, I had no fear of death—none at all. I'd just as soon have cuddled up down there beside her as not, and since that time I haven't had the least fear of death. I remember noticing at the time that the grave wasn't so very deep, and it sort of brought her home to me. Yet, when the coffin was being lowered into the grave, I wanted to holler, 'Stop!'"[28]

Heine, the poet, says explicitly that he would—nay, *will*— "cuddle up down there beside" his sweetheart, should she die:

Mein süsses Lieb, wenn du im Grab,
Im dunkeln Grab wirst liegen,
Dann will ich steigen zu dir hinab,
Und will mich an dich schmiegen.

Ich Küsse, umschlinge und presse dich wild,
Du Stille, du Kalte, du Bleiche!
Ich jauchze, ich zittre, ich weine mild,
Ich werde selber zur Leiche.[29]*

Poe says much the same thing:

For the moon never beams, without bringing me dreams
Of the beautiful Annabel Lee;
And the stars never rise, but I feel the bright eyes
Of the beautiful Annabel Lee.
And so, all the night-tide, I lie down by the side
Of my darling—my darling—my life and my bride,
In the sepulchre there by the sea—
In her tomb by the sounding sea.[30]

The suicidal impulse to restoration may be explicit. For example: "He resolved to die in this sorrow, having no other pleasure than that of following his child to the tomb."[31]

If the secondary belief in immortality is strong, there may be some such reaction as the following, in which the urge of the sorrow of love for restoration is quite as plain as in former examples:

Immortal, I feel it and know it,
Who doubts it of such as she?
But that is the pang's very secret,—
Immortal away from me.[32]

*My sweetest love, when you will bide,
In the grave and dark earth hold you,
I shall leap down to lie by your side,
Then shall my arms enfold you.

Wild, I will kiss you, I'll cling to your breast,
My still one, my cold one, pale lying.
Rejoicing, I tremble; soft weeping, I'm pressed
To your heart; I am dead in your dying.
                    Translated by E. Louise Mally

These illustrations sufficiently exemplify the principle that "the sorrow of love tends to restore that state of the beloved object, or that relation to it, the loss or destruction of which is the cause of the sorrow."

Principles 4, 5, and 6 below are in a way corollaries and recapitulations of what has preceded.

(4) Whenever the impulse of joy which maintains the state on which it is dependent is interrupted, so that the joy also is at an end, it tends to elicit an impulse to restore that state.[33]

(5) The absence, injury or destruction of an object of joy tends to arouse a type of sorrow which is distinguished by its impulse of restoration, and derives from the preceding joy an impulse of attraction to its object.[34]

(6) According as these impulses of attraction and restoration of sorrow are furthered, impeded, or frustrated, the emotion is itself diminished, increased or reaches its maximum.[35]

These principles state, in terms of arrested impulse, the cause of the types of sorrow described in principles 2 and 3. In one way or another, the *will-to-live* has met with a force stronger than itself, or one of its attendant wishes for response or recognition has been thwarted.

(7) The intensity of emotions is proportioned, other things being equal, to the degree in which they contrast with preceding or accompanying states.[36]

As a corollary:

(8) Sorrow tends to be increased by the close precedence of joy, and in proportion to the clearness of our remembrance of it in our experience; and again, by perceiving the signs of joy around us, and in a less degree by the thought that, while we sorrow, others rejoice.[37]

Thus, Dante says,

> No greater grief than to remember days
> Of joy, when misery is at hand.[38]

Another great poet repeats it:

> . . . a sorrow's crown of sorrows is remembering happier
> things.[39]

Many more illustrations of this same principle might be adduced
if space permitted.

> (9) Sorrow tends to be diminished by the close precedency and
> by the remembrance of other sorrow in our experience, and again by
> the perception of the signs of sorrow around us, and in some, though
> in a less degree, by the knowledge of such suffering.

A Spanish author observes: "One sorrow soothes another's
bitterness,"[40] and another says, "To think of bygone sorrows
soothes the troubles of today."[41] The working of this principle is
further shown by the fact that if the evil from which we suffer
seems peculiar to ourselves, or not fairly distributed in the world,
we are apt to have an angry feeling at its injustice. Here is one
aspect of the "problem of evil" about which so much Christian
theology centers. Men wonder why *they* seem singled out for misfortune, and like Job, curse their day and the Maker thereof. Some,
however, find comfort in the notion of a suffering Savior, bearing
perpetually the miseries and sins of the world. "Mythology tells
us that the Gods are not exempt from suffering; its aim, I suppose,
being to lighten our sorrow at death by the thought that even
deities are subject to it."[42] And "it is a consolation," says Seneca,
"to a humble man in trouble that the greatest are subject to
reverses of fortune, and a man weeps more calmly over his dead
son in the corner of his hovel, if he sees a piteous funeral proceed
out of the palace."[43] It was observable in the World War that, as
in the face of other shared disasters, the frequency of bereavement
was one factor in mitigating grief.

But when some sensitive soul ponders on the amount of misery
and grief about him, and thinks of its implications in terms of the
"problem of evil," the opposite may result, as in the following
example:

> That loss is common would not make
> My own less bitter, rather more.
> Too common! Never morning wore
> To evening, but some heart did break.[44]

This is a product of rational reflection, however, and not a primary emotional reaction, so that our principle stands unshaken.

(10) In proportion as the event which causes sorrow is both sudden and unexpected, it tends also to arouse surprise, and therefore to increase the intensity or strength of the sorrow.[45]

(11) In proportion as the event which causes sorrow either occurs gradually or is foreseen, the sorrow on that account tends to be felt with less intensity or strength.[46]

The two principles here stated are closely connected with 8 and 9.

Thus surprise renders it more difficult for bereaved individuals to bear up under the load—it is like dropping a heavy weight on the shoulders of a man who, if it were done gradually, would be quite able to bear it, but who is seriously strained because of the sudden shock. On the other hand, by breaking the news gradually, the method is like that of a street-car conductor who "feeds" his current by degrees in order to prevent "blowing" a fuse, or like the practice of giving serum injections in progressively increasing doses—each stimulus arouses a compensating resistance more able to withstand the next shock.

If, however, the attempt to forestall sorrow by foresight, which is akin to this "breaking the news gradually," becomes morbid brooding and foreboding, it is wasteful and may defeat its purpose, at least so far as net quantity of misery is concerned. Similarly, it is conceivable that a fixed habit of joy in life and its purposes, or even a routine, may carry an individual over a crisis of bereavement better than would prophetic "preparedness."

At first, the shock of surprise tends to confuse the mind so that a girl, for example, cannot realize that her mother is really dead. But when she has grasped the situation, her sorrow is nevertheless intensified by the original surprise. Sometimes, however, when the surprise is extreme, such persons do not recover from its effects. It is necessary, therefore, to take into account a limiting condition of the principle that surprise intensifies sorrow: the effect of surprise on the nervous system must not be so great as permanently to deprive the bereaved person of the degree of intelligence required to realize his misfortune.

(12) Sorrow tends to be diminished by the knowledge that another sorrows with us.[47]

(13) Sorrow tends to be increased by the knowledge that another rejoices at our suffering.[48]

> To weep with them that weep doth ease some deal,
> But sorrow flouted at is double death.[49]

Even the knowledge that others do not sorrow as greatly as we do produces these reactions, as the following excerpts show:

> Subject and sister felt very much isolated and alone. Felt that mourning by relatives not all sincere. No reasons for this; "just felt that way." This made subject also feel very bitter—why, did not know. Mourners all stood up about the casket, and one of them—subject did not remember which—made a few remarks, then nearest relatives took handles of casket and bore it out to waiting hearse. No songs or music of any sort. Nature of remarks made is not remembered; subject was consumed by sort of "dumb bitterness"; heard nothing that was said.
>
> Subject got some comfort out of presence of mourners, but on whole wished they would have stayed away; "we knew that most of them really weren't very sorry. Why, I don't believe that more than one or two of them cried!"[50]

This last remark furnishes an interesting contrast with the proverb:

> He gives little who gives tears,
> He gives much who aids and cheers.

> A principal fruit of friendship is the ease and discharge of the fullness and swellings of the heart. . . . Friendship works two contrary effects, for it redoubleth joys, and cutteth griefs in halves.[51]

Most attempts to account for the phenomena spoken of above make use of theories of sympathy. They do not satisfactorily explain them, however, because these theories leave out the disinterested element which changes the whole workings of the processes causing responses of a "sympathetic" nature.[52] What actually happens is this: Sorrow is the emotion of weakness, one affective factor in the wish for security. Its fundamental impulse is the appeal for help; and the knowledge that someone is willing to help us is a partial fulfillment of its appeal. On the other hand, the knowledge that when we are so weak our enemy is ready to take advantage of our weakness will tend to increase sorrow by obstructing the fulfillment of its impulse, the wish for security, and when anger is aroused in the service of this wish, sorrow becomes bitter, so to say.

(14) Sorrow tends to become more painful through being kept secret.[53]

(15) Sorrow tends to become less painful by being disclosed, so far as it seems to evoke pity in the recipient, or at least sympathetic emotion.[54]

> Give sorrow words: the grief that does not speak
> Whispers the o'erfraught heart, and bids it break.[55]

> Sorrow concealed, like an oven stopp'd,
> Doth burn the heart to cinders where it is.[56]

> Only the sorrow which keeps silence is more sad.[57]

> He oft finds med'cine who his griefe imparts.[58]

> So sorrow is cheered by being poured from one vessel
> to another.[59]

(16) Sorrow, like other painful states, becomes less painful and less intense when its emotion is controlled, and more painful and intense when uncontrolled.[60]

A distinction must be made, however, between that control of sorrow which consists in concealing it from others and the control of the emotion itself. The first, as already noted, increases it under certain conditions; the second diminishes it. Yet sorrow is often said to be relieved by tears and sighs because, sometimes at least, it works itself out in this way and comes to an end. There are those in whom it is intense but shallow, like the anger of the "touchy" or "irascible." In other cases, loss of self-control has not this compensating advantage.

The sorrow of the common people is ordinarily taciturn and patient, but sometimes it bursts into tears, into lamentation that seems ceaseless, above all those of the women. This sort of grief is no more easy to bear than the silent kind.[61]

The sort of relief which these lamentations produce is artificial and serves only to deepen the wound the heart has suffered, as one irritates an ulcer by touching it. It is a dolefulness that does not want consolation: it feeds upon itself.[62]

(17) Sorrow tends to arouse anger under opposition to its impulse, when the opposing force is not too strong and there is sufficient available energy to resist it.[63]

This principle connecting sorrow and anger is very difficult to limit and define because it really depends upon a quantity or degree of resistance which cannot be measured. There must be a ratio between the energy at our disposal and the resistance which thwarts our wishes for response, recognition, etc., before the arrested impulse of sorrow, or that of any other emotion, can excite anger. When the ratio is neither too great nor too small we have such instances as the following "temper-tantrum" poem:

> . . . that God for one so frail should form
> With clumsy cruelty—until you die—
> Peaks of sharp pain, I cannot and *I will*
> *Not understand,* but will *forever cry*
> Against all gods on Heaven's implacable hill,
> *Hoarding in ecstasy my hate and breath*
> To curse the sad incompetence of Death.[64]

Compare with this snatch of poetry the next illustration, which is a statement by an embittered girl with comment by her younger sister:

"There was an old woman, about eighty, in the hospital where Mother was. The very night Mother died, this old woman, who was so old that her mind was feeble, sat up in bed and began to whimper. I thought right then that a God that would take my mother, only forty-two years old, and leave that old woman alive, was not a God at all, even if He was [existed]. So I go to church no more." (Also ceased to believe in immortality, which was never believed in very strongly. Filled with sort of sullen anger against universe.)

"I never got angry at God that way Rebecca did—she used to make my blood run cold. I know that it's hard Mother was taken from us, but there was a reason for it, and it was a good reason. God does all things for the best. I was afraid Rebecca would go crazy after Mother died. She used to talk to herself and talk to God out loud, and if she had known then how to swear at Him, I believe she would have done it. She never knew I listened—she never said anything to me about it all, but kept it all inside her, although I used to try to get her to talk to me about it. I was afraid to tell her I knew some of the things she was thinking about."[65]

Milder, but still charged with bitterness:

One writes, that "other friends remain,"
That "loss is common to the race,"—
And common is the commonplace,
And vacant chaff well meant for grain.

Your logic, my friend, is perfect,
Your moral most drearily true;
But, since the earth clashed on *her* coffin,
I keep hearing that, and not you.

Console if you will, I can bear it,
'Tis a well-meant alms of breath:
But not all the preaching since Adam
Has made Death other than Death.[67]

Job soon became angry with the three friends who came to console him, and they passed the rest of their time together in recrimination.[68]

(18) Sorrow, whether caused by loss or destruction of an object of love, or by separation from it, or merely by the mood or temper, tends to destroy the belief in the intrinsic value of all other things previously valued.[69]

No fact is more conspicuous, or more amply illustrated in literature, than that sorrow tends to diminish and destroy the value which other sentiments attach to their objects. This is often referred to in metaphorical terms. The earth seems to be "darkened." Often the bereaved, for instance, can see nothing cheerful around them; they dress in black, and sit in darkened rooms. Occupations formerly pursued with energy and pleasure seem to lose interest,[70] to evoke repugnance, which reactions undoubtedly are largely due to ambivalence. Augustine thus describes his sorrow in youth at the death of a dear friend: "At this grief my heart was utterly darkened, and whatever I beheld was death. My native country was a torment to me, and my father's house a strange unhappiness; and whatever I had shared with him, wanting him, became a distracting torture. Mine eyes sought him everywhere . . . and I hated all places for that they had not him."[71] This excerpt shows a large element of ambivalence. Goethe, in describing the sorrow of Meister at the loss of Mariana, depicts the young poet and lover of the stage as treating with contempt his own talents, which he had before rated so highly.[72] Thus, through sorrow, the valuation which a man's egocentric tendency places upon himself may be destroyed like the value he places on other things; therefore, as has frequently been noted, sorrow lessens pride.

Several other principles are observable in the manifestations of sorrow in general, but Shand's analyses seem too fine-spun to be of much use in a social psychology of bereavement alone. They are cited below, however, without illustration or comment, for the sake of completeness. For bereavement, they represent an analysis and formulation of the tendency to concentrate on the lost one and to resist the reconditioning of affectional responses or the substitution of attachments.

(19) So far as the sorrow of love diminishes the valuation of things hitherto valued, and prevents one attaching a value for oneself to new things, it tends to increase the value attributed to its own object.[73]

(20) The sorrow of love tends to arouse repugnance, or disgust, or contempt for all objects that distract it from its own object and thereby strengthens itself.[74]

(21) Sorrow in distinction from joy contracts the mind to its object and is not attracted to other things; but it tends to make them objects of indifference or repugnance, and always of repugnance when they are thrust upon us and demand attention on their own account[75]

(22) When sorrow escapes from the perception or remembrance of its object it tends to become itself forgotten, and to be replaced by joy; but joy when it ceases to perceive or remember its object tends to be itself remembered, and, so far as it is referred to other objects, not to be replaced by sorrow.[76]

(23) The more the impulse of desire of sorrow becomes urgent and prominent in consciousness the more—other things equal—is the sorrow increased; the less prominent, the more is the sorrow diminished.[77]

This concludes the abstract, illustration, and interpretation of Shand's "laws of sorrow." They are, to be sure, more or less "rule of thumb" and empirical, for his psychological theory and method make altogether too much use of "instinct" and of introspection. Once having working hypotheses, however, no matter how vague, it may be possible to restate or reinterpret those hypotheses in more objective terms. The writer feels that this must be done if suggestions and recommendations for the lessening of the sorrows of bereavement are to be more than the well-meant platitudes they now are, and has attempted such interpretation here and there.

Now for a summary: (1) The marked difference in the "sorrow content" of preliterate behavior as reported by early observers and the written records and behavior of literate peoples was commented upon, and the suggestion made that perhaps the difference is not so great as it appears on the surface. (2) Reference was made to the validity of using literature as a basis for inductive psychological theorizing, and (3) the psychologist who has made the greatest use of such material, Shand, was mentioned and the assumptions or starting points of his own working hypotheses were outlined—primary instincts, emotions, etc. The provisional and tentative nature of his method was noted. A summary and abstract of his *Foundations of Character,* with interspersed comment and illustration by the writer, next occupied our attention, and (4) the four main types of sorrow were shown to owe their marked dissimilarities to the varying degrees of energy possessed by the organism and the varying strength of the sorrow stimulus, as well as to the intermixture of anger, fear, or other emotions. (5) The fact that sorrow is a consequence of the partial or complete frustration of some fundamental impulse or wish was next discussed. (6) The reasons for the characteristic behavior of sorrow were next analyzed, and the conclusion reached that such behavior has as its essential end the obtaining of help from others to remedy the weakness of the organism which cannot realize its thwarted wishes. (7) The peculiar attractive force of the sorrow of love was next stated, illustrated and commented upon, and the same method followed in the exposition of most of the other principles selected as of significance for this study. (8) A group of five principles were then cited without illustration because the writer felt that their importance, for the ends toward realization of which this study may prove of some preparatory help, was not great enough to warrant more elaborate treatment. Last of all, (9) the empirical and unscientific nature of these rule-of-thumb principles was pointed out, and the need for a more satisfactory method insisted upon.

NOTES

1. A. F. Shand, *The Foundations of Character* (London: Macmillan, second edition, 1920), Chapter X.
2. W. McDougall. *An Outline of Psychology* (London: Methuen, 1923), p. 9.
3. Shand, *op. cit.*, pp. vii–viii.
4. It should be noted that the present article is a highly condensed version of part of a lengthy unpublished study of the social psychology of bereavement. The original impetus that led to this study was due to Prof. T. D. Eliot of Northwestern University.
5. Spenser, *Faërie Queene.*
6. DeQuincey, *Suspiria de Profundis.*
7. E. B. Browning, "Grief."
8. Tennyson, *In Memoriam*, XX; 9–12.
9. Tennyson, "Home They Brought Her Warrior Dead," in the poem "The Princess," Part V.
10. Holmes, "The Voiceless," lines 17–18.
11. Masefield, "The Widow in the Bye Street," Part VI, septet 35, in *Poems and Plays of John Masefield* (New York: Macmillan, 1923), v. i., p. 245.
12. Lange, "La Tristesse," Les Emotions.
13. DeQuincey, "Our Ladies of Sorrow," in *Suspiria de Profundis.*
14. *King Lear*, Act I, Scene 5.
15. Cf. the following, from case studies made by the writer:

> "I was surprised at my own ability to keep going, especially as I had been under great strain just before I got news of the death. Then when this word came, I thought I'd break down, but I didn't. Surprised at myself."

> "Immediately after the death of his grandfather, subject got very little sleep. In spite of this fact, and in spite of additional fact that he is of frail physique, he felt himself buoyed up by an unusual access of strength — no feeling of weakness or unusual fatigue."

16. Shand, *op. cit.*, pp. 304–305.
17. Gray, *Letters,* quoted by Arnold, Chapt. "Gray," *Essays and Criticisms.*

18. Shand's "law" No. 58. Numbers hereafter given in notes are Shand's.

19. Shand, *op. cit.*, pp. 314–318.

20. No. 59.

21. Case study made by the writer.

22. Dickens, *David Copperfield*, Everyman's Library edition, Chap. iii, p. 37.

23. Tennyson, *op. cit.*, III and LIX.

24. *Ibid.*, I, lines 11–16.

25. *Ibid.*, XXVI, lines 1–4.

26. Case study by the writer.

27. No. 60.

28. Case study by the writer.

29. Heine, "Lyrisches Intermezzo," XXXII, 1–8; from *Buch der Lieder*, Insel edition, p. 105.

30. Poe, "Annabel Lee," 16th stanza.

31. Calvin, Institutio, 332, quoted by Littré, art. "Tristesse," *Dictionnaire*. (Translation by the writer.)

32. Lowell, "After the Burial," 7th stanza.

33. No. 61.

34. No. 62.

35. No. 63.

36. No. 64.

37. No. 65.

38. Dante, "Inferno," Canto V, lines 68–70, *The Divine Comedy*, Cary's translation.

39. Tennyson, "Locksley Hall."

40. Va yas-y-Ponce, quoted by Harbottle, *Dictionary of Quotations*, p. 37.

41. *Ibid.*, p. 49.

42. Seneca, "Epistolae," VI, 3.

43. Seneca, *op. cit.*, "De Ira," LIII, XXV.

44. Tennyson, *In Memoriam*, VI, 5–8.

45. No. 67.

46. No. 68.

47. No. 69.

48. No. 70.

49. Shakespeare, *Titus Andronicus*, Act III, Scene 1, lines 245-246.

50. Case studies made by the writer.

51. Bacon, "Of Friendship," Essays.

52. Cf. the writer's article: "Some Forms of Sympathy: A Phenomenological Analysis," *Journal of Abnormal and Social Psychology*, April 1931.

53. No. 71.

54. No. 72.

55. Shakespeare, *MacBeth*, Act IV, Scene 3.

56. Shakespeare, *Titus Andronicus*, Act II, Scene 5.

57. Racine, *Andromède*, III, 3.

58. Spenser, *Faërie Queene*, Bk. I, C. II, stanza xxxiv.

59. Hood, "Her Misery," Miss Killmansegg.

60. No. 73.

61. Dostoievsky, *The Brothers Karamazov*.

62. *Ibid.*

63. No. 75.

64. Harold Cook, "The Curse," last 7 lines, *Scrawl*, Northwestern University, April 1925, italics the writer's.

65. Case studies by the writer.

66. Tennyson, *op. cit.*, VI, 1–4.

67. Lowell, *op. cit.*, 8th and 9th stanzas.

68. The socializing effect of bereavement, with some temperaments, should be noted:

> "The shade by which my life was crost,
>   Which makes a desert in the mind,
>   Has made me kindly with my kind."
> Tennyson, *op. cit.*, LXVI, 5–8.

"'The captain had been struck dead by thundering apoplexy. It is a curious thing to understand, for I certainly had never liked the man, though of late I had begun to pity him, but as soon as I saw that he was dead, I burst into a flood of tears. It was the second death I had known, and the sorrow of the first was still fresh in my heart.'" Stevenson, *Treasure Island*, Everyman's Library edition, p. 18.

"... scholar Dick ... told him about his own father's death, which had happened when Dick was a child at Dublin, not quite five years of age. 'That was the first sensation of grief,' Dick said, 'I ever knew. I remember I went into the room where his body lay, and my mother sat weeping beside it. I had my battledore in my hand, and fell a-beating the coffin, and calling papa; on which my mother caught me in her arms, and told me in a flood of tears papa could not hear me, and would play with me no more ... And this,' said Dick kindly, 'has made me pity all children ever since; and caused me to love thee, my poor fatherless, motherless lad.'" Thackeray, *Henry Esmond*, Everyman's Library edition, p. 78.

69. No. 77.

70. "Aboulia" or lack of will to pursue other interests may be due to the absorption of energies in the bereavement conflict.

71. St. Augustine, *Confessions*, Bk. IV, 9.

72. Goethe, *Wilhelm Meister's Apprenticeship*, Bk. II, Chap. II (Carlyle's translation).

73. No. 80. This has a corollary No. 79: "Joy tends to form judgments which attribute intrinsic value to its object, when the intelligence is capable of forming them."

74. No. 81.

75. No. 82.

76. No. 81E.

77. No. 81F.

III. A SYMBOLIC ACTION DURING BEREAVEMENT

ROBERT F. CREEGAN

The bereavement situation has an intrinsic interest for the psychologist of human personality, because bereavement, in one form or another, intervenes as a decisive turning point in every life history. Specific cases may also have a secondary interest, for, like any severe crisis, the trauma of bereavement may bring to light many unsuspected characteristics of a personality which operate in veiled form at other times, also, in the life history.

This note presents a description and an analysis of a symbolic incident in the conduct of an adolescent male American under conditions of bereavement. This case, which I shall call "Our Little Joke," for reasons which will soon become clear, should help us understand the psychodynamics of the typical bereavement situation, although the case is unusual in certain respects. Its bizarre nature merely serves to exaggerate some very typical modes of response, but the study is also designed to explain some of the unique aspects of the personality involved.

The preliminary facts came to my attention in connection with my duties as a college instructor in philosophy. A certain young man exposed "Our Little Joke" in a term paper in aesthetics, which was supposed to be an essay concerning the category of the ugly. I will not embellish his story with the affective language of that colorful sophomore production. It concerned the death of an old dog (a decrepit terrier bitch) at the hands of its young master.

The first attempt at the avowedly "mercy killing" failed, because the high-school youth was inefficient in concocting potassium cyanide in the school laboratory and administered an ineffective dose. A few evenings later, as the youth sat in the poor and unattractive "den" of his home, observing the old dog's painful breathing, a compulsive idea that it must die at first annoyed and then overwhelmed him. In a highly emotional state, he devised a noose, and hung the animal from his own hands out of an open window. After half a minute, he dropped his struggling burden, and seizing a kitchen knife, administered the *coup de grace* with that instrument. This incident was called "Our Little Joke" by an exiled Scotsman, a chronic alcoholic, who, as janitor of the apartment, found the mangled body and inferred the circumstances. The janitor's term, "'Our Little Joke," was most consoling to the youth, removing the state of anxiety which had followed the action.

Both the story itself and the fact that it was told in a college term paper made some action on my part, as an instructor, necessary. I could not forget this sordid trifle, this "Little Joke," as I suspected that it was autobiographical and of clinical significance. I requested the youth to come to my office for an interview. A brilliant young man, much concerned with the ills of humanity, he had on more than one occasion in college life displayed aggressive tendencies of the sort that play such a large part in the Nazi-Fascist youth movements. But I found that his world panacea was quite as original a concoction as had been the potassium cyanide of the youth in his exposition. The first interview confirmed the conviction that the exposition was autobiographical. Subsequent interviews revealed the full circumstances. "Our Little Joke" happened a few days after the death of the youth's mother, when he was seventeen years old. Her heart attack concluded a political argument with the son. Just before the attack, she had said, as if begging for peace: "You are right, I have always known that you were right." Her death made him a complete orphan, as his father had died in an airplane crash years before. At the time of her death he admitted no grief or remorse but continued his scholastic and social activities as though nothing had happened.

The affective language of the youth's confession indicated that the events recorded in the paper were not simply historical. He was still deeply "involved," and the paper, itself an attempted catharsis, an attempted escape from "ego involvement," was also a means toward further relief. Far from evading the interviews, the youth welcomed them, and his deliberate resistance against making full confession were merely formal and very brief in duration. He sought a belated escape from grief and shock by such display. Exhibition of grief, with restraint, is typical of the bereavement situation, but the youth's initial reticence, followed a few years later by the exhibitions noted here, is, of course, atypical.

"Our Little Joke," as a deed, rather than as a story, was also typically motivated in a number of respects. The deed was an aggression. We have noted that aggression is a typical mode of response for our subject, but that particular aggression was in a situation which often provokes aggressive responses even from generally mild personalities. On one occasion in the interviews the youth gloatingly called his petty deed "my crime," and that, he admitted, was his original name for it. "Our Little Joke," the name offered by the exiled alcoholic, had been accepted with some relief as it made the aggression seem more trivial. But the old Scottish exile had, after all, appreciated the aggressive symbolism of the youth's deed, and that is why he called it "ours." The janitor was also bereaved, by circumstance, rather than by death, and he regarded the circumstance as unjust. The youth, often sympathetic in domestic relationships, did not feel that he had deserved his mother's passing-away during one of their rare disputes. Certain passages from the youth's diary indicate rather clearly that the "joke" was a retaliatory symbol. "Nothing cares," he wrote, at about that time. Other contemporaneous entries in the diary praise Nietzsche's philosophy of "ruthlessness." Nothing cares, therefore be ruthless; there is no cosmic justice, therefore aggress unjustly: This was the affective logic which motivated "Our Little Joke." But the general attitude is rather typical, bereavement is often interpreted animistically as a cosmic injustice.

Retaliation was one motive among many. The "joke" was symbolic on more than one level of affective meaning. The youth's distasteful academic exhibitionism in the paper, his enjoyment of the interviews, and the "joke" itself, all had obvious masochistic aspects. The "joke" was petty and sordid, and yet was done at a crucial juncture in the life history, at a time that would necessarily be remembered. Trivial in itself, memory of the deed would mean enduring shame, for the ego was, by that deed, irrevocably associated with the trivial and sordid. The youth's attitude toward this is illustrated by an oft-repeated dream of his, which is recorded in the diary, and which he says still recurs, although at increasing intervals. The dream is that his first offspring will be none other than a female terrier, much to the consternation of all concerned, and especially of the innocent prospective wife, who resembles the mother. The humor of the situation is not at all lost upon the youth, it partly compensates for his being haunted by a deed which he felt might so haunt him before he performed it. It was an attempt enduringly to injure himself, a self-inflicted punishment for his verbal aggression against the mother in the dispute which culminated in her heart attack and death. But remorse, during bereavement, is in itself typical.

At the same time, in the death of the bitch, the death of another dearly beloved old female was reenacted with "cathartic" effect, and it is also reenacted with masochistic concomitants in the occasional neurotic "heart attacks" which have subsequently been suffered by the youth. The "joke" expressed a "repetition compulsion," and was thus a means of resolving a psychic trauma.

In conclusion it may be said that the above description and analysis tend to show that both the episode which we have called "Our Little Joke," and our subject's later references to that episode, veiled and otherwise, express certain psychological "dynamisms" which, in their most general characteristics, are quite typical of bereavement situations and of attempts to resolve "tensions" which are engendered in such situations. As our above discussion heavily underscored each such typical "dynamism," as soon as it was revealed, the list of "dynamisms" need not be repeated here. Much that is atypical, and even bizarre, also appeared in this particular case, but most of its unusual features can be accounted for quite easily in terms of certain traits in our subject's personality. His rather high degree of insight, together with his very high affectivity, should be noted. These should be understood in their reciprocal relations: He seems to have used his self-knowledge, on more than one occasion, only as subservient to his symptoms, as a means of elaborating upon them. His was the poet's, rather than the scientific psychologist's, self-knowledge. These specific traits do not surprise us so much when we reflect that, in this case, we have been dealing with a spoiled only child of intelligent parents, whose home life after an early age was with a rather emotional mother. "Our Little Joke" has become for him a prime symbol of the conflict between ideality and reality, as this conflict is expressed in various phases of personal and social living. Any clinical intervention as late as the time at which this case came to the writer's attention could be expected at most only to keep his tendency to dramatize within limits of legal sanity. And, after all, most personal life quests, consciously lived as such, are expressed in certain prime symbols which are, in no few cases, quite as irrational as "Our Little Joke."

IV. REACTIONS TO
UNTIMELY DEATH

SAMUEL R. LEHRMAN

Scientific psychiatric interest in grief and other reactions to actual loss of a loved person through death stems from the psychoanalytic investigation of pathological depressions. Abraham,[1] in 1911, noted the similarity in psychic structure between manic-depressive depressions, involutional melancholia, and neurotic depressions, and was the first to point out the marked structural similarity of depressive psychosis to obsessional neurosis. Freud,[2] in 1916, amplified Abraham's observations in the classic paper "Mourning and Melancholia." He introduced the concept of mourning as a process, noted the similarity between mourning and melancholia, and was able to show the structural difference between the two conditions. "Mourning is regularly the reaction to the loss of a loved person or to the loss of some abstraction which has taken the place of one, such as fatherland, liberty, an ideal, and so on. As an effect of the same influences, melancholia, instead of a state of grief, develops in some people." Freud demonstrated that the psychopathology of melancholia revolved around introjection of the love object with a feeling of loss of love due to ambivalence and to sadistic attack on the introject.

Other writers have commented and enlarged on various aspects of Freud's work. Abraham[3] emphasized the pregenital stages of the libido in depressions, and introduced the concept of "primal depression." Rado[4] stressed the blows to narcissism, and endeavored to evolve the plan of interaction between the separate mental phenomena and their origin. He considered melancholia to be "a despairing cry for love" and postulated an "alimentary orgasm" which followed nursing. Melanie Klein's formulations[5] marked the "infantile depressive position" in the first year of life. There is a decided similarity to Freud, Abraham, and Rado, but she places the development of the psychic structures of the mind much earlier than they (first year of life), and considers the various "positions" to be self-preservative defensive measures. Gero,[6] and Jacobson[7] also stress the importance of disappointment in childhood, but underline the role of the oedipal conflict. Lewin,[8] in his brilliant book *The Psychoanalysis of Elation* has summarized the literature on depression and elation, and emphasized the "oral triad" in these conditions ("a wish to eat, a wish to be eaten—to enjoy a yielding relaxation—, and a wish to go to sleep").

Other authors, unlike the foregoing who were primarily interested in the manic-depressive conditions, have written of individual reactions to the death of a loved one. Helene Deutsch[9] described cases where the patients reacted to both timely and untimely death with "absence of grief." Charles Anderson[10] described pathological grief reactions among men suffering from war neuroses. Stern, Williams and Prados[11] described several "grief reactions in later life." Martin Peck[12] presented at length the case history of a forty-year-old man who developed a depression on learning of his wife's incurable illness, and whose psychoanalytic treatment extended over a period which included her death. Peck's patient presented a depressive reaction to untimely death. A. A. Brill[13] presented a case report of a man who reacted to the untimely death of his wife with a manic attack, following a mild depression.

The phrase "untimely death" refers to a death which occurs in a relatively young person. It also implies a disadvantageous timing in its occurrence. The death may be actual and sudden; or the pronouncement of incurability, serving as a death sentence, may usher in the reaction (cf. Peck's case). There is frequently surprise, shock and lack of preparation. On ordinary condolence calls, one inevitably hears the cliché: "When death occurs it is always a shock, no matter how well prepared you are." This is a conventional utterance with euphemistic, ego-defensive intent; it is not true. Grief reactions are actually much more normal when death occurs in an aged person and has been expected. Under such circumstances the work of mourning is done quickly, because a certain amount of this work (detaching the libido from the object) has already preceded the event of death. Pathological reactions to death are more frequent when the death is untimely and sudden. Other conditions also contribute to the formation of these pathological reactions.

The present paper is concerned with some variants of pathological reactions to untimely death, their origin, and meaning. The clinical material consists of five case histories. In two of the cases (Case 1 and Case 5) a young husband died suddenly of a heart attack. In one case, a thirty-year-old woman learned that her best friend had been found to have an incurable disease. In another, a mother lost her twenty-two-year-old son. In Case 4, a woman who came for treatment for a postpartum depression revealed the connections of this reaction with her reaction to her father's untimely death when she was four years old.

Case Material

CASE 1

A forty-year-old widow was seen in consultation at a general hospital. She had taken a bottle of "sleeping pills" and then had called her family doctor and told him about it. One year before, her husband had died suddenly of coronary thrombosis. She stated that she had "felt too shocked to cry" (absence of grief), but subsequently she felt lost. She felt very lonely and would often cry herself to sleep. She thought of suicide often, but was kept from action by a sense of responsibility to her three children. The estate left to her was small and she worked to supplement her income, but she was not happy working and sought marriage. A few weeks after the husband's funeral she began to go out on dates, but was distressed that middle-aged marriageable men were more interested in sex than in marriage. A widower with children proposed, but she considered the marriage impossible for "financial" reasons.

Her suicide attempt was a reaction of disappointment in her relations with another man. She had gone to his apartment in the course of establishing a permanent relationship with him, and was disturbed when he failed to call her during the following week. Her (oral) demanding expectations were characteristic of her relations with her husband, toward whom she had always felt ambivalent. Her castrative aggressiveness toward him was revealed in sexual frigidity and in interference with his business progress. She stated, "My husband has always been a passionate man, and I've always been an affectionate *man*" (the slip of the tongue further reveals penis envy). Her mother had come to live with her after her husband died, and this increased her super-ego and dependency conflicts. When she started to "date" at an age approaching forty, her social rustiness contributed to severe narcissistic injury. Her attitude toward the friend who was the occasion of the suicide attempt was similar to, and in some respects repeated, her attitude toward her husband. Her reaction to her husband's untimely death was close to one of "absence of grief," but the suicide attempt undoubtedly contains unresolved residuals of the reaction.

CASE 2

A thirty-five-year-old married woman, the mother of two children, was referred for psychiatric treatment because of a number of physical complaints for which no organic basis could be found. She presented a chief complaint of "I have pain." This pain occurred in the back, in the thoracic and lumbar regions. She said that it had started with an epigastric spasm approximately a month after she had learned that her best friend had an incurable disease. Her aging mother, too, had developed a chronic illness. The patient's history included an "ulcer spasm" about 12 years before, and a severe depression, with successful psychiatric treatment, about ten years before her present illness. She had had claustrophobia of varying severity since childhood. There were also compulsions and obsessions. Up to the time of her present illness she had made an excellent social adjustment, but with considerable anxiety. Her illness served the secondary gain of relieving social pressure; understandably she was much distressed if anyone commiserated with her.

Following a difficult pregnancy with her second child (sacroiliac strain, threatened abortion, and severe hemorrhoids), she was advised to avoid pregnancy. This proscription (=castration) called forth defensive measures against feelings of inferiority. She had always avoided contraceptive responsibility and the authoritative medical advice, added to her previous prudishness, justified increased reluctance to have sexual intercourse. Intercourse usually took place after an evening of "social" drinking. During the course of treatment, she blamed her husband for her difficulties, and she clung tenaciously to the position of a wronged wife.

This attitude had been carried over from childhood. Her mother had always been afraid of illness and of doctors, and had adopted an ostrich attitude when the children were sick, so that the patient was seriously neglected in childhood. Her friend's condition had been early misdiagnosed, and when the correct diagnosis was made, it was too late. The patient's attitude toward doctors, her husband and her friend contained much ambivalence with marked (repressed) aggression and identification originating in maternal transference. The actual death of the friend was of small significance, although the patient cried at the funeral. The conversion symptoms, connected as they were with identification and introjection, served the purpose of warding off a deep depression and possible suicide. They continue to be operative, but with decreasing intensity.

CASE 3

A forty-one-year-old married woman, the mother of three children, was referred for psychiatric treatment because of persistent pain in the right knee and leg. She presented as a chief complaint, "I haven't been the same since my son had his leg amputated." This had occurred about a year before her first visit, and she dreaded the approaching anniversary. The son had died six months after the operation and the patient experienced much grief (painful affect, loss of interest in the outside world and inability to love or be loved). However, she felt it necessary to withhold her tears at the funeral or when her family was watching, and she cried only in secret. When her aged father died, some time later, the patient said she could feel nothing.

The patient was the third of four children with immediately older and younger brothers. She had been brought up in a puritanical atmosphere and had married early, naïve and inexperienced. Her sex life was dull, but she soon became pregnant and was able to obtain great joy from identification with her son. (Conversely her daughters were a constant trouble.)

There were no overt phobias or obsessions, but the patient presented features of a mixed hysterical and compulsive character. She was perfectionistic, exacting and punctual, and had a need for affection and dramatic action. Her penis envy, disguised by reaction formation, appeared in her ambivalence toward husband, children and her career. She reacted to her son's leg amputation with conversion symptoms which warded off feelings of guilt linked to her aggression, the pain of penis envy, and grief over the loss of the son with whom she identified. The reaction formation of love for her son (carried over from her brothers) failed when he lost his leg. The narcissistic injury caused by symbolic castration increased her aggressions and guilt and doubled the ego-defensive burden of identification. These mechanisms continued after the son's death. Suicidal impulses appeared, and she could only react to her father's more timely death (which was insult added to injury) with absence of grief. This reaction was different from not crying at the son's funeral. There she defiantly (aggressively) displayed her "masculine" strength. The absence of grief was due to further regression. The conversion symptoms disappeared during treatment in which she was encouraged to cry and to share her grief with her husband. She discontinued treatment as the underlying neurotic character structure became exposed.

CASE 4

A twenty-six-year-old married woman was referred for treatment because of a postpartum depression. She had married against her mother's advice and had developed a markedly dependent attitude toward her mother-in-law. The birth of her son had aroused in her a considerable amount of latent sibling rivalry. (Although an only child, she had been a pupil in her mother's school class.) Further narcissistic injury resulted from the expectation of her mother-in-law that she care for her child. In the course of analysis the development of her obsessive-compulsive and depressive trends unfolded. Her mother, a schoolteacher, had toilet-trained her early, abandoned her to a housekeeper, and returned to work, but at the insistence of the father, a moderately successful engineer, had stopped working when the child was two years old.

The father had wanted a boy, but had been extremely affectionate until his death when the patient was four years old. The patient lost an important source of narcissistic supplies at the onset of the oedipal period, and the injury was compounded when her mother again returned to work, this time out of necessity. The patient sought to please her mother and other caretakers, and learned that she could keep her mother at home by becoming ill. She developed into a markedly obsessive-compulsive character with asthma, skin allergies and depressive trends. With considerable emotional conflicts, she competed successfully with the children in her mother's class and developed an attitude of overvaluation to money and intellect. To be wealthy meant that mother would love her, since mother paid more attention to the other (wealthy) children in the private school where she taught; this also meant that mother's approval was determined by her attitude toward feces during toilet-training. The patient's giving birth to her own child reactivated this complex (cf. the equation: child=feces=money[14]). The intellectual interests originating in oral and anal levels (identification with mother and *her* compulsiveness) were reinforced by penis envy at the oedipal level. The child reacted to her father's death with a repetition of her earlier response to loss of her mother, reinforcing the development of depressive and obsessional trends. This case represents a prime example of Abraham's early observation of the relations between depression and obsession-neurosis, and of Jacobson's observations[7] of the interrelatons of the Oedipus complex with depressions.

CASE 5

A twenty-seven-year-old married woman, the mother of two sons, presented a chief complaint of "I have an empty feeling, nothing to live for." She thought her difficulties had started about a month before her initial visit when her husband gave her a gold cupid for a charm bracelet as a birthday present. The patient did not realize the value of the gift and considered it to be a joke. This offended the husband and he showed his temper publicly. The patient said she "cried hysterically and felt something snap." Her immediate history is relevant to this reaction. Following an appendectomy, pulmonary embolism and subsequent miscarriage, she was told to avoid pregnancy (cf. Case 2) because of a tendency to thrombophlebitis. She craved a "tiny baby" and especially a daughter. The gold "baby" was, therefore, felt by her as a mockery, and the repressed anger burst through the censorship.

The patient had been the firstborn to undemonstrative, obsessional parents. She was brought up largely by "nurses" and maids. She resented the arrival of her siblings, but managed her hostility through partial repression and reaction formation. Although she was attractive and talented, her childhood and adolescence were unhappy. It was an achievement that she married the man she loved when she was nineteen. She disregarded her slight phobias and compulsiveness when they were uncovered during her treatment.

The patient improved under psychotherapy. She related to the therapist, and was able to verbalize, and accept, a small amount of hidden resentment toward her husband. Doubt was thrown on her magical beliefs (that she was being punished for past sins by being denied a third child) when her internist granted her permission to try to become pregnant. Two months after she became pregnant, at a time when discussion of terminating her treatment was taking place, her husband developed a benign subacute illness which confined him to bed for two months. During this time, the patient became obsessed with the idea that he would die and that she was being punished—partly for past misdeeds, and partly because this was her husband's way of disapproving of pregnancy. (The intimation of couvade could not be avoided. She said, "He always gets sick whenever I'm pregnant.")

A week after his recovery, while his six-months-pregnant wife was jubilantly planning a party to celebrate it, the man suddenly dropped dead. The patient was acutely shocked. She screamed and cried and then withdrew and denied the occurrence. She was heavily sedated and was seen by the writer on the following day. The reaction of apathy and denial continued. It was insisted that she attend the funeral, where she wept bitterly. During the mourning period which followed, she remained in bed, refused religious ministry or any other attempt at solace, but was not averse to being seen by the writer daily. She was withdrawn from her children, but was able after a few weeks to be up and about. She abjured cosmetics and ate poorly. Treatment was directed at encouraging her to grieve, with particular emphasis on the reality aspects of her situation.

Three months after her husband's death, she gave birth to a daughter. About a month after leaving the hospital, she gave up her home and moved her family to her parents' home. Her mother seemed understanding, but her father pressed her "to snap out of it." She continued with her psychotherapy, but became much attached to a woman relative slightly older than herself. She seemed to be working through the mourning, but received a marked setback from a relatively minor event. Her relative (mother surrogate) took a short vacation with her husband; the patient reacted to it as though she had once more been abandoned. She (again) stopped eating—with suicidal intent, and became more and more emaciated. Ambulatory insulin therapy at home and in a general hospital produced no particular effects. She began to talk about distortion in the size and appearance of her hands. After the writer had consulted with a colleague, about a week after admission to the hospital, electric convulsive therapy (ECT) was begun.

The administration of ECT was preceded by an intravenous injection of sodium amytal. As a consequence of the combined treatment the patient was able to sleep well for the first time in many weeks. Her reaction to the writer was interesting. She wanted to know "why Dr. Lehrman didn't give the treatment," and she greeted him by saying she "was mad" at him for not being present (even though he had been present). The meaning of this is clear when seen in the light of maternal transference. Although it seemed as if the patient had erotized the relationship to the writer in a genital way, this was not wholly the case. She was expressing anger at her mother for not taking care of her and was saying: "Mother [Dr. L.] should remain with me, feed me, nurse me and put me to sleep" (cf Lewin[8]). The distortion in hand size was related to her having been slapped by her piano teacher for "bad playing," and represented guilt over masturbation. Her reaction to her husband's untimely death was determined by her early relations with her mother, since her marriage relationship had been maintained largely on a pregenital level. She had carried over to her husband an ambivalent reaction formation (sibling rivalry), and an oral-anal dependency which originated in the infantile ambivalent attitude toward mother and caretakers. These feelings became obtrusive when she felt rejected by him. Her initial depressive reaction underwent further regression toward narcissistic withdrawal as a consequence of severe reality shocks which combined with the internal mechanisms to overwhelm the ego. A full course of ECT was disappointing in its results. After alternating periods of apathy and manic agitation, the patient was hospitalized in a distant city and gradually recovered.*

DISCUSSION

Reactions to untimely death may be considered to be variants of grief reactions. They differ from ordinary grief reactions in that the ego is less prepared for the loss, and in that the actual threat to the patient's ego is much greater. This external threat activates previously conditioned internal sadomasochistic impulses. Other conditions contributing to the formation of these patho-logical reactions are: previously existing psychopathology in the mourner, weakness of the ego, and absence of compensations in substitute love objects. Those patients who would tend to develop depressions (in the absence of death loss), or pathological grief reactions to expected or timely death, would inevitably develop pathological reactions to untimely death. It cannot be said, how-ever, that pathological reactions to untimely death are only depressions or depression equivalents, although prolonged dejec-tion often appears as part of the clinical picture. Conversion hys-teria is frequent enough to suggest one meaning for the heretofore confusing lay description of tears as "hysterical."

Even in situations of *timely* death, Helene Deutsch[9] has shown that when the ego feels threatened it may attempt to protect itself by absence of grief. (She feels, however, that ultimately the work of mourning must be done.) Her study confirms that of Freud, in ascribing great importance to the degree of persisting ambiva-lence and guilt feelings toward the lost love object. She gives as motives for exclusion of affect: (1) unendurability because of the ego's weakness—as in children, (2) submission to other claims of the ego, especially through narcissistic cathexis, (3) previously existing conflict with the lost object. She indicates that grief may take various forms, but her main thesis is that "the process of

---

*The mechanism of anorexia in this case may be compared to that described by Gero (Ref. 15). The writer has also observed obesity which developed in two adolescent girls as depression-equivalents in response to death of the father.

mourning as reaction to the real loss of a loved person must be carried to completion." Her patients, like those described in the present paper, reacted in accordance with their childhood conditioning, in further clinical confirmation of the genetic principle in psychoanalytic theory.

Anderson[10] studied 100 cases of morbid grief and classified the reactions in the following clinical patterns: anxiety states 59 percent, hysterias 19 percent, obsessional tension states 7 percent, and manic-depressive responses 15 percent. He observed that these reactions "were neither pure in type nor static," and that the clinical picture changed as the work of mourning proceeded. His case examples were all war neurotics who were themselves exposed to physical danger, and in some instances the patients actually killed the lost object (so that guilt was *not* merely in fantasy); thus the untimeliness of the loved one's death seemed to contribute nothing to the determination of the clinical pathology. Anderson's conclusions, however, coincide with Deutsch's and the present writer's: ". . . Certain neurotic responses are attempts to deal with and cure profound states of depression."

Stern, Williams and Prados[11] observe the following phenomena among "grief reactions in later life": an absence of grief, a preponderance of somatic illness, and a displaced irrational hostility toward living persons. While such reactions occasionally occur in younger persons subjected to untimely-death loss, the general characteristics described are more closely associated with advancing age in the mourner. It is to be noted, too, that these grief reactions were in response to the deaths of persons in later years, so that the deaths could not be considered untimely. In late middle age and particularly in old age, even when a death is sudden, there is a certain amount of preparation for it. A tentative explanation, advanced by the authors for these phenomena, is valid for the present paper: The assumption is that the symptoms are a "defense against dynamic forces that would be destructive to a weakened ego."

Lindemann[16] and Keeler[17] each write about grief reactions without discussing the dynamic importance of the untimeliness of the deaths in their cases. Lindemann's case material is largely based on reactions to accidental deaths in a nightclub fire. Many of his patients were participants in the tragic event; hence their reactions (like those described by Anderson) may have been parts of traumatic neuroses. Curiously, Lindemann cannot correlate the reactions to previous psychological status. Keeler studied 11 children's reactions to the death of a parent and notes in order of frequency: depression, fantasies of reunion, identification, delinquent behavior, suicidal attempts, and anxiety. He makes no attempt to explain the reactions, other than to liken them to normal and pathological mourning states. The writer has observed catatonic-like grief reactions with recovery in adolescents who have lost young parents. The young children in Case 5 of the present paper reacted with absence of grief. The mechanism of denial so frequently seen in depressions is also obtrusive in reactions to untimely death.

The similarity to traumatic neurosis of reactions to untimely death of a nonaccidental kind is marked. The need to master the psychological shock is common to both conditions. The mode of mastery determines the clinical picture, and is set by childhood patterning.*

That all the foregoing cases are women may be a coincidence (allowed by the small sampling; Peck's and Brill's patients were men), or may suggest that the incidence of these reactions—as in manic-depressive reactions—is higher in women than in men. (The part played by orality in determining depressive reactions has long been known.[1,2,3,8] Spitz[18] has emphasized the role of the mother. More recently Benedek,[19] and Engel and Reichsman[20] have written of a "biological depressive constellation." Clinically Fabian and Donohue[21] have called attention to the frequency of depressions in the mothers of clinic patients. Further discussion of depression not related to untimely death would be beyond the scope of this paper.)

In addition to the foregoing observations, the writer has had occasion to observe more closely several normal reactions to untimely death: the cases of parents who reacted with the usual manifestations of grief to death of a child by illness or accident. In all these instances, the factors of untimeliness were not threatening to the mourners' egos. This ego-sparing may have reduced the impact sufficiently to permit normal grief reactions. Other

*Dr. H. I. Schneer has called to the writer's attention the moving picture *Forbidden Games,* where children play a cemetery game in attempt at mastery.

factors contributing to the ego strength of the bereaved also played a part. In past times, when child death was common, parents were prepared through a state of almost constant expectation of death.

With reference to treatment, Freud[2] pointed out that in both mourning and melancholia, when the work of mourning is done, the patient automatically recovers. Deutsch[9] felt that there was only a temporary gain for the patient in displacement of affect. Lindemann[16] advised the conversion of abnormal grief into normal grief by sharing the patient's grief work. He was optimistic about recovery. For fear of precipitating psychosis, Anderson[10] warned against the use of physical or chemical means to produce quick abreaction. He felt that ECT, as in other types of reactive depression, was valueless. The writer's experience suggests that while reactions to untimely death should be treated as variants of grief reactions, they tend to be refractory, and patients are likely to be in therapy for a long time.

Varying conditions determine the ultimate prognosis (which was fairly good in the writer's cases). ECT in Case 5 prevented the formation of further somatic delusions, but had little effect on the manic agitation and none on the overall clinical picture. Psycho-analysis, when feasible (Case 4), reveals the underlying structure of the neurosis and permits control of the affect experienced by the patient. (Kaufman[22] is optimistic about this procedure even in late life depressions.) Where suicide is a serious threat, hospitalization may be advisable. In treatment by psychotherapy (Cases 2, 3, 5), ambivalence in the transference should be watched for, and the patient should have adequate opportunity for the expression of affect in appropriate doses.

Summary and Conclusions

From the literature and the writer's clinical material, the following conclusions are drawn:

1. Reactions to untimely death are variants of pathological grief and mourning, and may assume the form of obsessive-compulsive neurosis, anxiety state, hysteria, manic-depressive psychosis, or schizoid state. The clinical pictures are usually mixed and atypical in accordance with the varying basic etiological factors. A similar-

ity to traumatic neurosis is present. A normal reaction may occur where ego strength is sufficient.

Where the reaction to untimely death is a pathological one, the clinical picture is determined by the patient's childhood conditioning, and the extent to which the infantile neurosis has been mastered. If there is an actual threat to the patient's ego (for example, loss of provider or caretaker), the trauma is more keenly felt. However, as in other psychiatric conditions, the (internal) fantasy trauma is more important than the actual one.

3. Reactions to untimely death tend to follow the pattern of grief reactions which represent a defense against unbearable, painful affect, or a defense against serious internal ego threat such as suicide.

4. Treatment should proceed slowly. Where drugs are employed, they should be sedative rather than abreacting. ECT is indicated only at the threat of, or in the presence of, psychosis. When the underlying infantile neurosis can be worked through, as in psychoanalysis, the prognosis is good, but psychoanalysis may not necessarily be the treatment of choice. In psychotherapy, the dosage of affect should be controlled. While it is true that completion of the work of mourning offers the best hope for successful outcome, a permanent neurotic compromise may be the best result obtainable in some cases.

REFERENCES

1. ABRAHAM, KARL. "Notes on the Psychoanalytical Investigation and Treatment of Manic-Depressive Insanity and Allied Conditions." In: *Selected Papers of Karl Abraham*. London: Hogarth Press and the Institute of Psychoanalysis, 1927.
2. FREUD, SIGMUND. "Mourning and Melancholia." In: *Collected Papers*, IV. London: Hogarth Press and the Institute of Psychoanalysis, 1924.
3. ABRAHAM, KARL. "A Short Study of the Development of the Libido Viewed in the Light of Mental Disorders." In: *Selected Papers of Karl Abraham*. London: Hogarth Press and the Institute of Psychoanalysis, 1927.
4. RADO, SANDOR. "The Problem of Melancholia." *Int. J. Psychoan.*, 9 (1928), p. 420.
5. KLEIN, MELANIE. "A Contribution to the Psychogenesis of Manic-Depressive States." In: *Contributions to Psychoanalysis 1921–1945*. London: Hogarth Press and the Institute of Psychoanalysis, 1948.
6. GERO, GEORGE. "The Construction of Depression." *Int. J. Psychoan.* 17 (1936).

7. JACOBSON, EDITH. "Depression–the Oedipus Conflict in the Development of Depressive Mechanisms." *Psychoan. Quart.,* 12 (1943), p. 541.

8. LEWIN, BERTRAM D. *The Psychoanalysis of Elation.* New York: Norton, 1950.

9. DEUTSCH, HELENE. "Absence of Grief." *Psychoan. Quart.,* 6 (1937), p. 12.

10. ANDERSON, CHARLES. "Aspects of Pathological Grief and Mourning." *Int. J. Psychoan.* 30 (1949), p. 48.

11. STERN, K., WILLIAMS, G., and PRADOS, M. "Grief Reactions in Later Life." *Am. J. Psychiat.* 108 (October 1951), p. 289.

12. PECK, MARTIN W. "Notes on Identification in a Case of Depression Reactive to Death of a Love Object." *Psychoan. Quart.,* 8 (1939), p. 1.

13. BRILL, A. A. "Mourning, Melancholia and Compulsions." In: *Yearbook of Psychoanalysis,* I. New York: International Universities Press, 1945.

14. FREUD, SIGMUND. "On the Transformation of Instincts with Special Reference to Anal Erotism. In: *Collected Papers,* II. London: Hogarth Press and the Institute of Psychoanalysis, 1924.

15. GERO, GEORGE. "An Equivalent of Depression: Anorexia." In: *Affective Disorders.* Phyllis Greenacre, editor. New York: International Universities Press, 1953.

16. LINDEMANN, ERICH. "Symptomatology and Management of Acute Grief." *Am. J. Psychiat.,* 101 (September 1944), p. 141.

18. SPITZ, RENE. "Anaclitic Depression. In: *The Psychoanalytic Study of the Child.* Vol. 2, 1946. New York: International Universities Press, 1947.

19. BENEDEK, THERESE F. "Toward the Biology of the Depressive Constellation." *J. Am. Psychoan. Asso.,* 4 (July 1956), p. 389.

20. ENGEL, GEORGE L., and REICHSMAN, FRANZ. "Spontaneous and Experimentally Induced Depression in an Infant with Gastric Fistula: A Contribution to the Problem of Depression." *J. Am. Psychoan. Asso.,* 4 (July 1956), p. 428.

21. FABIAN, A. A., and DONOHUE, JOHN F. "Maternal Depression: A Challenging Child Guidance Problem." *Am. J. Orthopsychiat,* 26 (April 1956), p. 400.

22. KAUFMAN, M. RALPH. "Psychoanalysis in Late Life Depressions." *Psychoan. Quart.,* 6 (July 1937), p. 308.

V. MOURNING AND ITS RELATION TO MANIC-DEPRESSIVE STATES

MELANIE KLEIN

An essential part of the work of mourning is, as Freud points out in "Mourning and Melancholia," the testing of reality. He says that "in grief this period of time is necessary for detailed carrying out of the behest imposed by the testing of reality, and ... by accomplishing this labour the ego succeeds in freeing its libido from the lost object."[1] And again: "Each single one of the memories and hopes which bound the libido to the object is brought up and hyper-cathected, and the detachment of the libido from it accomplished. Why this process of carrying out the behest of reality bit by bit, which is in the nature of a compromise, should be so extraordinarily painful is not at all easy to explain in terms of mental economics. It is worth noting that this pain seems natural to us."[2] And, in another passage: "We do not even know by what economic measures the work of mourning is carried through; possibly, however, a conjecture may help us here. Reality passes **its** verdict—that the object no longer exists—upon each single one of the memories and hopes through which the libido was attached to the lost object, and the ego, confronted as it were with the decision whether it shall share this fate, is persuaded by the sum of its narcissistic satisfactions in being alive to sever its attachment to the non-existent object. We may imagine that, because of the slowness and the gradual way in which this severance is achieved, the expenditure of energy necessary for it becomes somehow dissipated by the time the task is carried through."[3]

In my view there is a close connection between the testing of reality in normal mourning and early processes of the mind. My contention is that the child goes through states of mind compar-

237

able to the mourning of the adult, or rather, that this early mourning is revived whenever grief is experienced in later life. The most
important of the methods by which the child overcomes his states
of mourning, is, in my view, the testing of reality; this process,
however, as Freud stresses, is part of the work of mourning.

In my paper "A Contribution to the Psychogenesis of Manic-
Depressive States,"⁴ I introduced the conception of the *infantile
depressive position* and showed the connection between that position and manic-depressive states. Now in order to make clear the
relation between the infantile depressive position and normal
mourning I must first briefly refer to some statements I made in
that paper, and shall then enlarge on them. In the course of this
exposition I also hope to make a contribution to the further understanding of the connection between normal mourning, on the one
hand, and abnormal mourning and manic-depressive states, on the
other.

I said there that the baby experiences depressive feelings which
reach a climax just before, during and after weaning. This is the
state of mind in the baby which I termed the "depressive position,"
and I suggested that it is a melancholia in *statu nascendi*. The
object which is being mourned is the mother's breast and all that
the breast and the milk have come to stand for in the infant's
mind: namely, love, goodness and security. All these are felt by the
baby to be lost, and lost as a result of his own uncontrollable greedy
and destructive fantasies and impulses against his mother's breasts.
Further distress about impending loss (this time of both parents)
arises out of the oedipus situation, which sets in so early and in
such close connection with breast frustrations that in its beginnings
it is dominated by oral impulses and fears. The circle of loved
objects who are attacked in fantasy, and whose loss is therefore
feared, widens owing to the child's ambivalent relations to his
brothers and sisters. The aggression against fantasied brothers and
sisters, who are attacked inside the mother's body, also gives rise
to feelings of guilt and loss. The sorrow and concern about the
feared loss of the "good" objects, that is to say, the depressive position, is, in my experience, the deepest source of the painful conflicts
in the oedipus situation, as well as in the child's relations to people
in general. In normal development these feelings of grief and fears
are overcome by various methods.

Along with the child's relation, first to his mother and soon to his father and other people, go those processes of internalization on which I have laid so much stress in my work. The baby, having incorporated his parents, feels them to be live people inside his body in the concrete way in which deep unconscious fantasies are experienced—they are, in his mind, "internal" or "inner" objects, as I have termed them. Thus an inner world is being built up in the child's unconscious mind, corresponding to his actual experiences and the impressions he gains from people and the external world, and yet altered by his own fantasies and impulses. If it is a world of people predominantly at peace with each other and with the ego, inner harmony, security and integration ensue.

There is a constant interaction between anxieties relating to the "external" mother—as I will call her here in contrast to the "internal" one—and those relating to the "internal" mother, and the methods used by the ego for dealing with these two sets of anxieties are closely interrelated. In the baby's mind, the "internal" mother is bound up with the "external" one, of whom she is a "double," though one which at once undergoes alterations in his mind through the very process of internalization; that is to say, her image is influenced by his fantasies, and by internal stimuli and internal experiences of all kinds. When external situations which he lives through become internalized—and I hold that they do, from the earliest days onwards—they follow the same pattern: they also become "doubles" of real situations, and are again altered for the same reasons. The fact that by being internalized, people, things, situations and happenings—the whole inner world which is being built up—becomes inaccessible to the child's accurate observation and judgment, and cannot be verified by the means of perception which are available in connection with the tangible and palpable object-world, has an important bearing on the fantastic nature of this inner world. The ensuing doubts, uncertainties and anxieties act as a continuous incentive to the young child to observe and make sure about the external object-world,[5] from which this inner world springs, and by these means to understand the internal one better. The visible mother thus provides continuous proofs of what the "internal" mother is like, whether she is loving or angry, helpful or revengeful. The extent to which external reality is able to disprove anxieties and sorrow relating to the internal reality varies with each indivdual, but could be taken as one of the criteria for normality. In children who are so much dominated by their internal world that their anxieties cannot be sufficiently disproved and counteracted even by the pleasant aspects of their relationships with people, severe mental difficulties are unavoidable. On the other hand, a certain amount even of unpleasant experiences is of value in this testing of reality by the child if, through overcoming them, he feels that he can retain his objects as well as their love for him and his love for them, and thus preserve or reestablish internal life and harmony in face of dangers.

All the enjoyments which the baby lives through in relation to his mother are so many proofs to him that the loved object *inside as well as outside* is not injured, is not turned into a vengeful person. The increase of love and trust, and the diminishing of fears through happy experiences, help the baby step by step to overcome his depression and feeling of loss (mourning). They enable him to test his inner reality by means of outer reality. Through being loved and through the enjoyment and comfort he has in relation to people his confidence in his own as well as in other people's goodness becomes strengthened, his hope that his "good" objects and his own ego can be saved and preserved increases, at the same time as his ambivalence and acute fears of internal destruction diminish.

Unpleasant experiences and the lack of enjoyable ones, in the young child, especially lack of happy and close contact with loved people, increase ambivalence, diminish trust and hope and confirm anxieties about inner annihilation and external persecution; moreover they slow down and perhaps permanently check the beneficial processes through which in the long run inner security is achieved.

In the process of acquiring knowledge, every new piece of experience has to be fitted into the patterns provided by the psychic reality which prevails at the time; whilst the psychic reality of the child is gradually influenced by every step in his progressive knowledge of external reality. Every such step goes along with his more and more firmly establishing his inner "good" objects, and is used by the ego as a means of overcoming the depressive position.

In other connections I have expressed the view that every infant experiences anxieties which are psychotic in content,[6] and that the infantile neurosis[7] is the normal means of dealing with and modifying these anxieties. This conclusion I can now state more precisely, as a result of my work on the infantile depressive position, which has led me to believe that it is the central position in the child's development. In the infantile neurosis the early depressive position finds expression, is worked through and gradually overcome; and this is an important part of the process of organization and integration which, together with the sexual development,[8] characterizes the first years of life. Normally the child passes through the infantile neurosis, and among other achievements arrives step by step at a good relation to people and to reality. I hold that this satisfactory relation to people depends upon his having succeeded in his struggles against the chaos inside him (the depressive position) and having securely established his "good" internal objects.

Let us now consider more closely the methods and mechanisms by which this development comes about.

In the baby, processes of introjection and projection, since they are dominated by aggression and anxieties which reinforce each other, lead to fears of persecution by terrifying objects. To such fears are added those of losing his loved objects; that is to say, the depressive position has arisen. When I first introduced the concept of the depressive position, I put forward the suggestion that the introjection of the whole loved object gives rise to concern and sorrow lest that object should be destroyed (by the "bad" objects and the id), and that these distressed feelings and fears, in addition to the paranoid set of fears and defenses, constitute the depressive position. There are thus two sets of fears, feelings and defenses, which, however varied in themselves and however intimately linked together, can, in my view, for purposes of theoretical clearness, be isolated from each other. The first set of feelings and fantasies are the persecutory ones, characterized by fears relating to the destruction of the ego by internal persecutors. The defenses against these fears are predominantly the destruction of the persecutors by violent or secretive and cunning methods. With these fears and defenses I have dealt in detail in other contexts. The second set of feelings which go to make up the depressive position I formerly described without suggesting a term for them. I now propose to use for these feelings of sorrow and concern for the loved objects, the fears of losing them and the longing to regain them, a simple word derived from everyday language—namely the "pining" for the loved object. In short—persecution (by "bad" objects) and the characteristic defenses against it, on the one hand, and pining for the loved ("good") object, on the other, constitute the depressive position.

When the depressive position arises, the ego is forced (in addition to earlier defenses) to develop methods of defense which are essentially directed against the "pining" for the loved object. These are fundamental to the whole ego-organization. I formerly termed some of these methods *manic defenses,* or the *manic position,* because of their relationship to the manic-depressive illness.[9]

The fluctuations between the depressive and the manic position are an essential part of normal development. The ego is driven by depressive anxieties (anxiety lest the loved objects as well as itself should be destroyed) to build up omnipotent and violent fantasies, partly for the purpose of controlling and mastering the "bad," dangerous objects, partly in order to save and restore the loved ones. From the very beginning these omnipotent fantasies, both the destructive and the reparative ones, stimulate and enter into all the activities, interests and sublimations of the child. In the infant the extreme character both of his sadistic and of his constructive fantasies is in line with the extreme frightfulness of his persecutors—and, at the other end of the scale, the extreme perfection of his "good" objects.[10] Idealization is an essential part of the manic position and is bound up with another important element of that position, namely denial. Without partial and temporary denial of psychic reality the ego cannot bear the disaster by which it feels itself threatened when the depressive position is at its height. Omnipotence, denial and idealization, closely bound up with ambivalence, enable the early ego to assert itself to a certain degree against its internal persecutors and against a slavish and perilous dependence upon its loved objects, and thus to make further advances in development. I will here quote a passage from my former paper [p. 308]:

> In the earliest phase the persecuting and the good objects (breasts) are kept wide apart in the child's mind. When, along with the introjection of the whole and real object, they come closer together, the ego has over and over again recourse to that mechanism—so important for the development of the relations to objects—namely, a splitting of its imagos into loved and hated, that is to say, into good

and dangerous ones.

One might think that it is actually at this point that ambivalence which, after all, refers to object-relations—that is to say, to whole and real objects—sets in. Ambivalence, carried out in a splitting of the imagos, enables the young child to gain more trust and belief in its real objects and thus in its internalized ones—to love them more and to carry out in an increasing degree its fantasies of restoration of the loved object. At the same time the paranoid anxieties and defenses are directed toward the "bad" objects. The support which the ego gets from a real "good" object is increased by a flight-mechanism, which alternates between its external and internal good objects. [Idealization.]

It seems that at this stage of development the unification of external and internal, loved and hated, real and imaginary objects is carried out in such a way that each step in the unification leads again to a renewed splitting of the imagos. But as the adaptation to the external world increases, this splitting is carried out on planes which gradually become increasingly nearer and nearer to reality. This goes on until love for the real and the internalized objects and trust in them are well established. Then ambivalence, which is partly a safeguard against one's own hate and against the hated and terrifying objects will in normal development again diminish in varying degrees.[11]

As has already been stated, omnipotence prevails in the early fantasies, both the destructive and the reparative ones, and influences sublimations as well as object relations. Omnipotence, however, is so closely bound up in the unconscious with the sadistic impulses with which it was first associated that the child feels again and again that his attempts at reparation have not succeeded, or will not succeed. His sadistic impulses, he feels, may easily get the better of him. The young child, who cannot sufficiently trust his reparative and constructive feelings, as we have seen, resorts to manic omnipotence. For this reason, in an early stage of development the ego has not adequate means at its disposal to deal efficiently with guilt and anxiety. All this leads to the need in the child—and for that matter to some extent in the adult also—to repeat certain actions obsessionally (this, in my view, is part of the repetition compulsion);[12] or—the contrasting method—omnipotence and denial are resorted to. When the defenses of a manic nature fail (defenses in which dangers from various sources are in an omnipotent way denied or minimized) the ego is driven alternately or simultaneously to combat the fears of deterioration and disintegration by attempted reparations carried out in obsessional ways. I have described elsewhere[13] my conclusion that the obsessional mechanisms are a defense against paranoid anxieties as well as a means of modifying them, and here I will only show briefly the connection between obsessional mechanisms and manic defenses in relation to the depressive position in normal development.

The very fact that manic defenses are operating in such close connection with the obsessional ones contributes to the ego's fear that the reparation attempted by obsessional means has also failed. The desire to control the object, the sadistic gratification of overcoming and humiliating it, of getting the better of it, the *triumph* over it, may enter so strongly into the act of reparation (carried out by thoughts, activities or sublimations) that the "benign" circle started by this act becomes broken. The objects which were to be restored change again into persecutors, and in turn paranoid fears are revived. These fears reinforce the paranoid defense mechanisms (of destroying the object) as well as the manic mechanisms (of controlling it or keeping it in suspended animation, and so on). The reparation which was in progress is thus disturbed or even nullified—according to the extent to which these mechanisms are activated. As a result of the failure of the act of reparation, the ego has to resort again and again to obsessional and manic defenses.

When in the course of normal development a relative balance between love and hate is attained, and the various aspects of objects are more unified, then also a certain equilibrium between these contrasting and yet closely related methods is reached, and their intensity is diminished. In this connection I wish to stress the importance of *triumph,* closely bound up with contempt and omnipotence, as an element of the manic position. We know the part rivalry plays in the child's burning desire to equal the achievements of the grown-ups. In addition to rivalry, his wish, mingled with fears, to "grow out" of his deficiencies (ultimately to overcome his destructiveness and his bad inner objects and to be able to control them) is an incentive to achievements of all kinds. In my experience, the desire to reverse the child-parent relation, to get power over the parents and to triumph over them, is always to some extent associated with desires directed to the attainment of success. A time will come, the child fantasies, when he will be strong, tall and grown up, powerful, rich and potent, and father and mother will have changed into helpless children, or again, in other fantasies, will be very old, weak, poor and rejected. The triumph over the parents in such fantasies, through the guilt to which it gives rise, often cripples endeavours of all kinds. Some people are obliged to remain unsuccessful, because success always implies to them the humiliation or even the damage of somebody else, in the first place the triumph over parents, brothers and sisters. The efforts by which they seek to achieve something may be of a highly constructive nature, but the implicit triumph and the ensuing harm and injury done to the object may outweigh these purposes, in the subject's mind, and therefore prevent their fulfilment. The effect is that the reparation to the loved objects, which in the depths of the mind are the same as those over which he triumphs, is again thwarted, and therefore guilt remains unrelieved. The subject's triumph over his objects necessarily implies to him their wish to triumph over him, and therefore leads to distrust and feelings of persecution. Depression may follow, or an increase in manic defenses and more violent control of his objects, since he has failed to reconcile, restore, or improve them, and therefore feelings of being persecuted by them again have the upper hand. All this has an important bearing on the infantile depressive position and the ego's success or failure in overcoming it. The triumph over his internal objects which the young child's ego controls, humiliates and tortures is a part of the destructive aspect of the manic position which disturbs reparation and re-creating of his inner world and of internal peace and harmony; and thus triumph impedes the work of early mourning.

To illustrate these developmental processes let us consider some features which can be observed in hypomanic people. It is characteristic of the hypomanic person's attitude toward people, principles and events that he is inclined to exaggerated valuations: overadmiration (idealization) or contempt (devaluation). With this goes his tendency to conceive of everything on a large scale, to think in *large numbers,* all this in accordance with the greatness of his omnipotence, by which he defends himself against his fear of losing the one irreplaceable object, his mother, whom he still mourns at bottom. His tendency to minimize the importance of details and small numbers, and a frequent casualness about details and contempt of conscientiousness contrast sharply with the very meticulous methods, the concentration on the smallest things (Freud), which are part of the obsessional mechanisms.

This contempt, however, is also based to some extent on denial. He must deny his impulse to make extensive and detailed reparation because he has to deny the cause for the reparation; namely, the injury to the object and his consequent sorrow and guilt.

Returning to the course of early development, we may say that every step in emotional, intellectual and physical growth is used by the ego as a means of overcoming the depressive position. The child's growing skills, gifts and arts increase his belief in the psychic reality of his constructive tendencies, in his capacity to master and control his hostile impulses as well as his "bad" internal objects. Thus anxieties from various sources are relieved, and this results in a diminution of aggression and, in turn, of his suspicions of "bad" external and internal objects. The strengthened ego, with its greater trust in people, can then make still further steps toward unification of its imagos—external, internal, loved and hated—and toward further mitigation of hatred by means of love, and thus to a general process of integration.

When the child's belief and trust in his capacity to love, in his reparative powers and in the integration and security of his good inner world increase as a result of the constant and manifold proofs and counterproofs gained by the testing of external reality, manic omnipotence decreases and the obsessional nature of the impulses toward reparation diminishes, which means in general that the infantile neurosis has passed.

We have now to connect the infantile depressive position with normal mourning. The poignancy of the actual loss of a loved person is, in my view, greatly increased by the mourner's unconscious fantasies of having lost his *internal* "good" objects as well. He then feels that his internal "bad" objects predominate and his inner world is in danger of disruption. We know that the loss of a loved person leads to an impulse in the mourner to reinstate the lost loved object in the ego (Freud and Abraham). In my view, however, he not only takes into himself (reincorporates) the person whom he has just lost, but also reinstates his internalized good objects (ultimately his loved parents), who became part of his inner world from the earliest stages of his development onwards. These too are felt to have gone under, to be destroyed, whenever the loss of a loved person is experienced. Thereupon the early depressive position, and with it anxieties, guilt and feelings of loss and grief derived from the breast situation, the oedipus situation and from all other sources, are reactivated. Among all these emotions, the fears of being robbed and punished by both dreaded parents—that is to say, feelings of persecution—have also been revived in deep layers of the mind.

If, for instance, a woman loses her child through death, along with sorrow and pain her early dread of being robbed by a "bad" retaliating mother is reactivated and confirmed. Her own early aggressive fantasies of robbing her mother of babies gave rise to fears and feelings of being punished, which strengthened ambivalence and led to hatred and distrust of others. The reinforcing of feelings of persecution in the state of mourning is all the more painful because, as a result of an increase in ambivalence and distrust, friendly relations with people, which might at that time be so helpful, become impeded.

The pain experienced in the slow process of testing reality in the work of mourning thus seems to be partly due to the necessity, not only to renew the links to the external world and thus continuously to reexperience the loss, but at the same time and by means of this to rebuild with anguish the inner world, which is felt to be in danger of deteriorating and collapsing.[14] Just as the young child passing through the depressive position is struggling, in his unconscious mind, with the task of establishing and integrating his inner world, so the mourner goes through the pain of re-establishing and reintegrating it.

In normal mourning early psychotic anxieties are reactivated. The mourner is in fact ill, but because this state of mind is common and seems so natural to us, we do not call mourning an illness. (For similar reasons, until recent years, the infantile neurosis of the normal child was not recognized as such.) To put my conclusions more precisely: I should say that in mourning the subject goes through a modified and transitory manic-depressive state and overcomes it, thus repeating, though in different circumstances and with different manifestations, the processes which the child normally goes through in his early development.

The greatest danger for the mourner comes from the turning of his hatred against the lost loved person himself. One of the ways in which hatred expresses itself in the situation of mourning is in feelings of triumph over the dead person. I refer in an earlier part of this paper to triumph as part of the manic position in infantile development. Infantile death-wishes against parents, brothers and sisters are actually fulfilled whenever a loved person dies, because he is necessarily to some extent a representative of the earliest important figures, and therefore takes over some of the feelings pertaining to them. Thus his death, however shattering for other reasons, is to some extent also felt as a victory, and gives rise to triumph, and therefore all the more to guilt.

At this point I find that my view differs from that of Freud, who stated: "First, then: in normal grief too the loss of the object is undoubtedly surmounted, and this process too absorbs all the energies of the ego while it lasts. Why then does it not set up the economic condition for a phase of triumph after it has run its course or at least produce some slight indication of such a state? I find it impossible to answer this objection off-hand."[15] In my experience, feelings of triumph are inevitably bound up even with normal mourning, and have the effect of retarding the work of mourning, or rather they contribute much to the difficulties and pain which the mourner experiences. When hatred of the lost loved object in its various manifestations gets the upper hand in the mourner, this not only turns the loved lost person into a persecutor, but shakes the mourner's belief in his good inner objects as well. The shaken belief in the good objects disturbs most painfully the process of idealization, which is an essential intermediate step in mental development. With the young child, the idealized mother is the safeguard against a retaliating or a dead mother and against all bad objects, and therefore represents security and life itself. As we know, the mourner obtains great relief from recalling the lost person's kindness and good qualities, and this is partly due to the reassurance he experiences from keeping his loved obect for the time being as an idealized one.

The passing states of elation[16] which occur between sorrow and distress in normal mourning are manic in character and are due to the feeling of possessing the perfect loved object (idealized) inside. At any time, however, when hatred against the lost loved person wells up in the mourner, his belief in him breaks down and the process of idealization is disturbed. (His hatred of the loved person is increased by the fear that by dying the loved one was seeking to inflict punishment and deprivation upon him, just as in the past he felt that his mother, whenever she was away from him and he wanted her, had died in order to inflict punishment and deprivation upon him.) Only gradually, by regaining trust in external obects and values of various kinds, is the normal mourner able once more to strengthen his confidence in the lost loved person. Then he can again bear to realize that this object was not perfect, and yet not lose trust and love for him, nor fear his revenge. When this stage is reached, important steps in the work of mourning and toward overcoming it have been made.

To illustrate the ways in which a normal mourner reestablished connections with the external world I shall now give an instance. Mrs. A., in the first few days after the shattering loss of her young son, who had died suddenly while at school, took to sorting out letters, keeping his and throwing others away. She was thus unconsciously attempting to restore him and keep him safe inside herself, and throwing out what she felt to be indifferent, or rather hostile— that is to say, the "bad" objects, dangerous excreta and bad feelings.

Some people in mourning tidy the house and rearrange furniture, actions which spring from an increase of the obsessional mechanisms which are a repetition of one of the defenses used to combat the infantile depressive position.

In the first week after the death of her son she did not cry much, and tears did not bring her the relief which they did later on. She felt numbed and closed up, and physically broken. It gave her some relief, however, to see one or two intimate people. At this stage Mrs. A., who usually dreamed every night, had entirely stopped dreaming because of her deep unconscious denial of her actual loss. At the end of the week she had the following dream: She saw two people, a mother and son. The mother was wearing a black dress. The dreamer knew that this boy had died, or was going to die. No sorrow entered into her feelings, but there was a trace of hostility toward the two people.

The associations brought up an important memory. When Mrs. A. was a little girl, her brother, who had difficulties in his schoolwork, was going to be tutored by a schoolfellow of his own age (I will call him B). B's mother had come to see Mrs. A.'s mother to arrange about the coaching, and Mrs. A. remembered this incident with very strong feelings. B's mother behaved in a patronizing way, and her own mother appeared to her to be rather dejected. She herself felt that a fearful disgrace had fallen upon her very much admired and beloved brother and the whole family. This brother, a few years older than herself, seemed to her full of knowledge, skill and strength—a paragon of all the virtues, and her ideal was shattered when his deficiencies at school came to light. The strength of her feelings about this incident as being an irreparable misfortune, which persisted in her memory, was, however, due to her unconscious feelings of guilt. She felt it to be the fulfillment of her own harmful wishes. Her brother himself was very much chagrined by the situation, and expressed great dislike and hatred of the other boy. Mrs. A. at the time identified herself strongly with him in these resentful feelings. In the dream, the two people whom Mrs. A saw were B and his mother, and the fact that the boy was dead expressed Mrs. A.'s early death wishes against him. At the same time, however, the death wishes against her own brother and the wish to inflict punishment and deprivation upon her mother through the loss of her son—very deeply repressed wishes—were part of her dream thoughts. It now appeared that Mrs. A., with all her admiration and love for her brother, had been jealous of him on various grounds, envying his greater knowledge, his mental and physical superiority, and also his possession of a penis. Her jealousy of her much beloved mother for possessing such a son had contributed toward her death wishes against her brother. One dream-thought, therefore, ran: "A mother's son has died, or will die. It is this unpleasant woman's son, who hurt my mother and brother, who should die." But in deeper layers, the death-wish against her brother had also been reactivated, and this dream-thought ran: "My mother's son died, and not my own." (Both her mother and her brother were in fact already dead.) Here a contrasting feeling came in—sympathy with her mother and sorrow for herself. She felt: "One death of the kind was enough. My mother lost her son; she should not lose her grandson also." When her brother died, besides great sorrow, she unconsciously felt triumph over him, derived from her early jealousy and hatred, and corresponding feelings of guilt.

She had carried over some of her feelings for her brother into her relation to her son. In her son, she also loved her brother; but at the same time, some of the ambivalence towards her brother, though modified through her strong motherly feelings, was also transferred on to her son. The mourning for her brother, together with the sorrow, the triumph and the guilt experienced in relation to him, entered into her present grief, and was shown in the dream.

Let us now consider the interplay of defenses as they appeared in this material. When the loss occurred, the manic position became reinforced, and denial in particular came especially into play. Unconsciously, Mrs. A. strongly rejected the fact that her son had died. When she could no longer carry on this denial so strongly—but was not yet able to face the pain and sorrow—triumph, one of the other elements of the manic position, became reinforced. "It is not at all painful," the thought seemed to run, as the associations showed, "if *a* boy dies. It is even satisfactory. Now I get my revenge against this unpleasant boy who injured my brother." The fact that triumph over her brother had also been revived and strengthened became clear only after hard analytic work. But this triumph was associated with control of the *internalized* mother and brother, and triumph over them. At this stage the *control* over her internal objects was reinforced, the misfortune and grief were *displaced* from herself on to her internalized mother. Here denial again came into play—denial of the psychical reality that she and her internal mother were one and suffered together. Compassion and love for the internal mother were denied, feelings of revenge and triumph over the internalized objects and control of them were reinforced, partly because, through her own revengeful feelings, they had turned into persecuting figures.

In the dream there was only one slight hint of Mrs. A.'s growing unconscious knowledge (indicating that the denial was lessening) that it was she *herself* who lost her son. On the day preceding the dream she was wearing a black dress with a white collar. The woman in the dream had something white round her neck on her black dress.

Two nights after this dream she dreamt again: She was flying with her son, and he disappeared. She felt that this meant his death —that he was drowned. She felt as if she, too, were to be drowned—

but then she made an effort and drew away from the danger, back to life.

The associations showed that in the dream she had decided that she would not die with her son, but would survive. It appeared that even in the dream she felt that it was good to be alive and bad to be dead. In this dream the unconscious knowledge of her loss is much more accepted than in the one of two days earlier. Sorrow and guilt had drawn closer. The feeling of triumph had apparently gone, but it became clear that it had only diminished. It was still present in her satisfaction about remaining alive—in contrast to her son's being dead. The feelings of guilt which already made themselves felt were partly due to this element of triumph.

I am reminded here of the passage in Freud's "Mourning and Melancholia":[17] "Reality passes its verdict—that the object no longer exists—upon each single one of the memories and hopes through which the libido was attached to the lost object, and the ego, confronted as it were with the decision whether it will share this fate, is persuaded by the sum of its narcissistic satisfactions in being alive to sever its attachment to the non-existent object." In my view, this "narcissistic satisfaction" contains in a milder way the element of triumph which Freud seemed to think does not enter into normal mourning.

In the second week of her mourning Mrs. A. found some comfort in looking at nicely situated houses in the country, and in wishing to have such a house of her own. But this comfort was soon interrupted by bouts of despair and sorrow. She now cried abundantly, and found relief in tears. The solace she found in looking at houses came from her rebuilding her inner world in her fantasy by means of this interest and also getting satisfaction from the knowledge that other people's houses and good objects existed. Ultimately this stood for re-creating her good parents, internally and externally, unifying them and making them happy and creative. In her mind she made reparation to her parents for having, in fantasy, killed their children, and by this she also averted their wrath. Thus her fear that the death of her son was a punishment inflicted on her by retaliating parents lost in strength, and also the feeling that her son frustrated and punished her by his death was lessened. The diminution of hatred and fear in this way allowed the sorrow itself to come out in full strength. Increase of distrust and fears had intensified her feeling of being persecuted and mastered by her internal objects and strengthened her need to master them. All this had expressed itself by a hardening in her internal relationships and feelings—that is to say, in an increase in manic defenses. (This was shown in the first dream.) If these again diminish through the strengthening of the subject's belief in goodness—his own and others'—and fears decrease, the mourner is able to surrender fully to his feelings, and to cry out his sorrow about the actual loss.

It seems that the processes of projecting and ejecting, which are closely connected with giving vent to feelings, are held up in certain stages of grief by an extensive manic control, and can again operate more freely when that control relaxes. Through tears, the mourner not only expresses his feelings and thus eases tension, but, since in the unconscious they are equated to excrements, he also expels his "bad" feelings and his "bad" objects, and this adds to the relief obtained through crying. This greater freedom in the inner world implies that the internalized objects, being less controlled by the ego, are also allowed more freedom: that these objects themselves are allowed, in particular, greater freedom of feeling. In the mourner's state of mind, the feelings of his internal objects are also sorrowful. In his mind, they share his grief, in the same way as actual kind parents would. The poet tells us that "Nature mourns with the mourner." I believe that "Nature" in this connection represents the internal good mother. This experience of mutual sorrow and sympathy in internal relationships, however, is again bound up with external ones. As I have already stated, Mrs. A.'s greater trust in actual people and things, and help received from the external world, contributed to a relaxing of the manic control over her inner world. Thus introjection (as well as projection) could operate still more freely, more goodness and love could be taken in from without, and goodness and love increasingly experienced within. Mrs. A., who at an earlier stage of her mourning had to some extent felt that her loss was inflicted on her by revengeful parents, could now in fantasy experience the sympathy of these parents (dead long since), their desire to support and to help her. She felt that they also suffered a severe loss and shared her grief, as they would have done had they lived. In her internal world harshness and suspicion had diminished, and sorrow had increased. The tears which she shed were also to some extent the tears which her internal parents shed, and she also wanted to comfort them as they—in her fantasy—comforted her.

If greater security in the inner world is gradually regained, and feelings and inner objects are therefore allowed to come more to life again, re-creative processes can set in, and hope return.

As we have seen, this change is due to certain movements in the two sets of feelings which make up the depressive position: persecution decreases and the pining for the lost loved object is experienced in full force. To put it in other words: hatred has receded and love is freed. It is inherent in the feeling of persecution that it is fed by hatred and at the same time feeds hatred. Furthermore, the feeling of being persecuted and watched by internal "bad" objects, with the consequent necessity for constantly watching them, leads to a kind of dependence which reinforces the manic defenses. These defenses, in so far as they are used predominantly against persecutory feelings (and not so much against the pining for the loved object), are of a very sadistic and forceful nature. When persecution diminishes, the hostile dependence on the object, together with hatred, also diminishes, and the manic defenses relax. The pining for the lost loved object also implies dependence on it, but dependence of a kind which becomes an incentive to reparation and preservation of the object. It is creative because it is dominated by love, while the dependence based on persecution and hatred is sterile and destructive.

Thus while grief is experienced to the full and despair is at its height, the love for the object wells up and the mourner feels more strongly that life inside and outside will go on after all, and that the lost loved object can be preserved within. At this stage in mourning, suffering can become productive. We know that painful experiences of all kinds sometimes stimulate sublimations, or even bring out quite new gifts in some people, who may take to painting, writing or other productive activities under the stress of frustrations and hardships. Others become more productive in a different way—more capable of appreciating people and things, more tolerant in their relation to others—they become wiser. Such enrichment is in my view gained through processes similar to those steps in mourning which we have just investigated. That is to say, any pain caused by unhappy experiences, whatever their nature, has something in common with mourning. It reactivates the infantile depressive position; the encountering and overcoming of adversity of any kind entails mental work similar to mourning.

It seems that every advance in the process of mourning results in a deepening in the individual's relation to his inner objects, in the happiness of regaining them after they were felt to be lost ("Paradise Lost and Regained"), in an increased trust in them and love for them because they proved to be good and helpful after all. This is similar to the ways in which the young child step by step builds up his relations to external objects, for he gains trust not only from pleasant experiences, but also from the ways in which he overcomes frustrations and unpleasant experiences, nevertheless retaining his good objects (externally and internally). The phases in the work of mourning when manic defenses relax and a renewal of life inside sets in, with a deepening in internal relationships, are comparable to the steps which in early development lead to greater independence from external as well as internal objects.

To return to Mrs. A. Her relief in looking at pleasant houses was due to the setting in of some hope that she could re-create her son as well as her parents; life started again inside herself and in the outer world. At this time she could dream again and unconsciously begin to face her loss. She now felt a stronger wish to see friends again, but only one at a time and only for a short while. These feelings of greater comfort, however, again alternated with distress. (In mourning as well as in infantile development, inner security comes about not by a straightforward movement but in waves.) After a few weeks of mourning, for instance, Mrs. A. went for a walk with a friend through the familiar streets, in an attempt to reestablish old bonds. She suddenly realized that the number of people in the street seemed overwhelming, the houses strange and the sunshine artificial and unreal. She had to retreat into a quiet restaurant. But there she felt as if the ceiling were coming down, and the people in the place became vague and blurred. Her own house suddenly seemed the only secure place in the world. In analysis it became clear that the frightening indifference of these people was reflected from her internal objects, who in her mind had turned into a multitude of "bad" persecuting objects. The external world was felt to be artificial and unreal, because real trust in inner goodness had temporarily gone.

Many mourners can only make slow steps in reestablishing the bonds with the external world because they are struggling against the chaos inside; for similar reasons the baby develops his trust in the object-world first in connection with a few loved people. No doubt other factors as well, e.g., his intellectual immaturity, are partly responsible for this gradual development in the baby's object relations, but I hold that this is also due to the chaotic state of his inner world.

One of the differences between the early depressive position and normal mourning is that when the baby loses the breast or bottle, which has come to represent to him a "good," helpful, protective object inside him, and experiences grief, he does this even though his mother is there. With the grown-up person, however, the grief is brought about by the actual loss of an actual person; yet help comes to him against this overwhelming loss through his having established in his early life his "good" mother inside himself. The young child, however, is at the height of his struggles with fears of losing her internally and externally, for he has not yet succeeded in establishing her securely inside himself. In this struggle, the child's relation to his mother, her actual presence, is of the greatest help. Similarly, if the mourner has people whom he loves and who share his grief, and if he can accept their sympathy, the restoration of the harmony in his inner world is promoted, and his fears and distress are more quickly reduced.

Having described some of the processes which I have observed at work in mourning and in depressive states, I wish now to link up my contribution with the work of Freud and Abraham.

Based on Freud's and his own discoveries about the nature of the archaic processes at work in melancholia, Abraham found that such processes also operate in the work of normal mourning. He concluded that in this work the individual succeeds in establishing the lost loved person in his ego, while the melancholic has failed to do so. Abraham also described some of the fundamental factors upon which that success or failure depends.

My experience leads me to conclude that, while it is true that the characteristic feature of normal mourning is the individual's setting up the lost loved object inside himself, he is not doing so for the first time but, through the work of mourning, is reinstating that object as well as all his loved *internal* objects which he feels he has lost. He is therefore *recovering* what he had already attained in childhood.

In the course of his early development, as we know, he establishes his parents within his ego. (It was the understanding of the processes of introjection in melancholia and in normal mourning which, as we know, led Freud to recognize the existence of the suger-ego in normal development.) But, as regards the nature of the super-ego and the history of its individual development, my conclusions differ from those of Freud. As I have often pointed out, the processes of introjection and projection from the beginning of life lead to the institution inside ourselves of loved and hated objects, who are felt to be "good" and "bad," and who are interrelated with each other and with the self: that is to say, they constitute an inner world. This assembly of internalized objects becomes organized, together with the organization of the ego, and in the higher strata of the mind it becomes discernible as the super-ego. Thus, the phenomenon which was recognized by Freud, broadly speaking, as the voices and the influence of the actual parents established in the ego is, according to my findings, a complex object-world, which is felt by the individual, in deep layers of the unconscious, to be concretely inside himself, and for which I and some of my colleagues therefore use the term "internalized objects" and an "inner world." This inner world consists of innumerable objects taken into the ego, corresponding partly to the multitude of varying aspects, good and bad, in which the parents (and other people) appeared to the child's unconscious mind throughout various stages of his development. Further, they also represent all the real people who are continually becoming internalized in a variety of situations provided by the multitude of ever-changing external experiences as well as fantasied ones. In addition, all these objects are in the inner world in an infinitely complex relation both with each other and with the self.

If I now apply this description of the super-ego organization, as compared with Freud's super-ego, to the process of mourning, the nature of my contribution to the understanding of this process becomes clear. In normal mourning the individual reintrojects and reinstates, as well as the actual lost person, his loved parents who are felt to be his "good" inner objects. His inner world, the one which he has built up from his earliest days onwards, in his fantasy was destroyed when the actual loss occurred. The rebuilding of this inner world characterizes the successful work of mourning.

An understanding of this complex inner world enables the analyst to find and resolve a variety of early anxiety-situations which were formerly unknown, and is therefore theoretically and therapeutically of an importance so great that it cannot yet be fully estimated. I also believe that the problem of mourning can only be more fully understood by taking account of these early anxiety situations.

I shall now illustrate in connection with mourning one of these anxiety-situations which I have found to be of crucial importance also in manic-depressive states. I refer to the anxiety about the internalized parents in destructive sexual intercourse; they as well as the self are felt to be in constant danger of violent destruction. In the following material I shall give extracts from a few dreams of a patient, D, a man in his early forties, with strong paranoid and depressive traits. I am not going into details about the case as a whole, but am here concerned only to show the ways in which these particular fears and fantasies were stirred in this patient by the death of his mother. She had been in failing health for some time, and was, at the time to which I refer, more or less unconscious.

One day in analysis, D spoke of his mother with hatred and bitterness, accusing her of having made his father unhappy. He also referred to a case of suicide and one of madness which had occurred in his mother's family. His mother, he said, had been "muddled" for some time. Twice he applied the term "muddled" to himself and then said: "I know you are going to drive me mad and then lock me up." He spoke about an animal being locked up in a cage. I interpreted that his mad relative and his muddled mother were now felt to be inside himself, and that the fear of being locked up in a cage partly implied his deeper fear of containing these mad people inside himself and thus of going mad himself. He then told me a dream of the previous night: He saw a bull lying in a farmyard. It was not quite dead, and looked very uncanny and dangerous. He was standing on one side of the bull, his mother on the other. He escaped into a house, feeling that he was leaving his mother behind in danger and that he should not do so; but he vaguely hoped that she would get away.

To his own astonishment, my patient's first association to the dream was of the blackbirds which had disturbed him very much by waking him up that morning. He then spoke of buffaloes in America, the country where he was born. He had always been interested in them and attracted by them when he saw them. He now said that one could shoot them and use them for food, but that they are dying out and should be preserved. Then he mentioned the story of a man who had been kept lying on the ground, with a bull standing over him for hours, unable to move for fear of being crushed. There was also an association about an actual bull on a friend's farm; he had lately seen this bull, and he said it looked ghastly. This farm had associations for him by which it stood for his own home. He had spent most of his childhood on a large farm his father owned. In between, there were associations about flower seeds spreading from the country and taking root in town gardens. D saw the owner of this farm again the same evening and urgently advised him to keep the bull under control. (D had learnt that the bull had recently damaged some buildings on the farm.) That very evening the patient received the news of his mother's death.

In the following hour, D did not at first mention his mother's death, but expressed his hatred of me—my treatment was going to kill him. I then reminded him of the dream of the bull, interpreting that in his mind his mother had become mixed up with the attacking bull-father—half-dead himself—and had become uncanny and dangerous. I myself and the treatment were at the moment standing for this combined parent-figure. I pointed out that the recent increase of hatred against his mother was a defense against his sorrow and despair about her approaching death. I referred to his aggressive fantasies by which, in his mind, he had changed his father into a dangerous bull which would destroy his mother; hence his feeling of responsibility and guilt about this impending disaster. I also referred to the patient's remark about eating buffaloes, and explained that he had incorporated the combined parent-figure and so felt afraid of being crushed internally by the bull. Former material had shown his fear of being controlled and attacked internally by dangerous beings, fears which had resulted among other things in his taking up at times a very rigid and immobile posture. His story of the man who was in danger of being crushed by the bull, and who was kept immobile and controlled by it, I interpreted as a representation of the dangers by which he felt threatened internally.[18]

I now showed the patient the sexual implications of the bull's attacking his mother, connecting this with his exasperation about the birds waking him that morning (this being his first association to the bull-dream). I reminded him that in his associations birds often stood for people, and that the noise the birds made—a noise to which he was quite accustomed—represented to him the dangerous sexual intercourse of his parents, and was so unendurable on this particular morning because of the bull-dream, and owing to his acute state of anxiety about his dying mother. Thus his mother's death meant to him her being destroyed by the bull inside him, since—the work of mourning having already started—he had internalized her in this most dangerous situation.

I also pointed out some hopeful aspects of the dream. His mother might save herself from the bull. Blackbrids and other birds he is actually fond of. I showed him also the tendencies to reparation and re-creation present in the material. His father (the buffaloes) should be preserved, ie., protected against his—the patient's—own greed. I reminded him, among other things, of the seeds which he wanted to spread from the country he loved to the town, and which stood for new babies being created by him and by his father as a reparation to his mother—these live babies being also a means of keeping her alive.

It was only *after* this interpretation that he was actually able to tell me that his mother had died the night before. He then admitted, which was unusual with him, his full understanding of the internalization processes which I had interpreted to him. He said that after he had received the news of his mother's death he felt sick, and that he thought, even at the time, that there could be no physical reason for this. It now seemed to him to confirm my interpretation that he had internalized the whole imagined situation of his fighting and dying parents.

During this hour he had shown great hatred, anxiety and tension, but scarcely any sorrow; toward the end, however, after my interpretation, his feelings softened, some sadness appeared, and he experienced some relief.

The night after his mother's funeral, D dreamt that X (a father-figure) and another person (who stood for me) were trying to help him, but actually he had to fight for his life against us; as he put it: "Death was claiming me." In this hour he again spoke bitterly about his analysis as disintegrating him. I interpreted that he felt the helpful external parents to be at the same time the fighting, disintegrating parents, who would attack and destroy him—the half-dead bull and the dying mother inside him—and that I myself and analysis had come to stand for the dangerous people and happenings inside himself. That his father was also internalized by him as dying or dead was confirmed when he told me that at his mother's funeral he had wondered for a moment whether his father was not also dead. (In reality the father was still alive.)

Toward the end of this hour, after a decrease of hatred and anxiety, he again became more cooperative. He mentioned that the day before, looking out of the window of his father's house into the garden and feeling lonely, he disliked a jay he saw on a bush. He thought that this nasty and destructive bird might possibly interfere with another bird's nest with eggs in it. Then he associated that he had seen, some time previously, bunches of wild flowers thrown on the ground—probably picked and thrown away by children. I again interpreted his hatred and bitterness as being in part a defense against sorrow, loneliness and guilt. The destructive bird, the destructive children—as often before—stood for himself who had, in his mind, destroyed his parents' home and happiness and killed his mother by destroying her babies inside her. In this connection his feelings of guilt related to his *direct* attacks in fantasy on his mother's body; whilst in connection with the bull-dream the guilt was derived from his *indirect* attacks on her, when he changed his father into a dangerous bull who was thus carrying into effect his—the patient's—own sadistic wishes.

On the third night after his mother's funeral, D had another dream:

He saw a bus coming toward him in an uncontrolled way—apparently driving itself. It went toward a shed. He could not see what happened to the shed, but knew definitely that the shed "was going to blazes." Then two people, coming from behind him, were opening the roof of the shed and looking into it. D did not "see the point of their doing this," but they seemed to think it would help.

Besides showing his fear of being castrated by his father through a homosexual act which he at the same time desired, this dream expressed the same internal situation as the bull-dream—the death of his mother inside him and his own death. The shed stood for his mother's body, for himself, and also for his mother inside him. The dangerous sexual intercourse represented by the bus destroying the shed happened in his mind to his mother as well as to himself; but in addition, and that is where the predominant anxiety lay, to his mother *inside* him.

His not being able to see what happened in the dream indicated that in his mind the catastrophe was happening internally. He also knew, without seeing it, that the shed was "going to blazes." The bus "coming toward him," besides standing for sexual intercourse and castration by his father, also meant "happening inside him."[19]

The two people opening the roof from behind (he had pointed to my chair) were himself and myself, looking into his inside and into his mind (psychoanalysis). The two people also meant myself as the "bad" combined parent-figure, myself containing the dangerous father—hence his doubts whether looking into the shed (analysis) could help him. The uncontrolled bus represented also himself in dangerous sexual intercourse with his mother, and expressed his fears and guilt about the badness of his own genitals. Before his mother's death, at a time when her fatal illness had already begun, he accidentally ran his car into a post—without serious consequences. It appeared that this was an unconscious suicidal attempt, meant to destroy the internal "bad" parents. This accident also represented his parents in dangerous sexual intercourse inside him, and was thus an acting out as well as an externalization of an internal disaster.

The fantasy of the parents combined in "bad" intercourse—or rather, the accumulation of emotions of various kinds, desires, fears and guilt, which go with it—had very much disturbed his relation to both parents, and had played an important part not only in his illness but in his whole development. Through the analysis of these emotions referring to the actual parents in sexual intercourse, and particularly through the analysis of these internalized situations, the patient became able to experience real mourning for his mother. All his life, however, he had warded off the depression and sorrow about losing her, which were derived from his infantile depressive feelings, and had denied his very great love for her.

Unconsciously he had reinforced his hatred and feelings of persecution, because he could not bear the fear of losing his *loved* mother. When his anxieties about his own destructiveness decreased and confidence in his power to restore and preserve her became strengthened, persecution lessened and love for her came gradually to the fore. But together with this he increasingly experienced the grief and longing for her which he had repressed and denied from his early days onward. While he was going through this mourning with sorrow and despair, his deeply buried love for his mother came more and more into the open, and his relation to both parents altered. On one occasion he spoke of them, in connection with a pleasant childhood memory, as "my dear old parents"—a new departure in him.

I have shown here and in my preceding paper the deeper reasons for the individual's incapacity to overcome successfully the infantile depressive position. Failure to do so may result in depressive illness, mania or paranoia. I pointed out *(op. cit.)* one or two other methods by which the ego attempts to escape from the sufferings connected with the depressive position, namely either the flight to internal good objects (which may lead to severe psychosis) or the flight to external good objects (with the possible outcome of neurosis). There are, however, many ways, based on obsessional, manic and paranoid defenses, varying from individual to individual in their relative proportion, which in my experience all serve the same purpose, that is, to enable the individual to escape from the sufferings connected with the depressive position. (All these methods, as I have pointed out, have a part in normal development also.) This can be clearly observed in the analyses of people who fail to experience mourning. Feeling incapable of saving and securely reinstating their loved objects inside themselves, they must turn away from them more than hitherto and therefore deny their love for them. This may mean that their emotions in general become more inhibited; in other cases it is mainly feelings of love which become stifled and hatred is increased. At the same time, the ego uses various ways of dealing with paranoid fears (which will be the stronger the more hatred is reinforced) . For instance, the internal "bad" objects are manically subjugated, immobilized and at the same time denied, as well as strongly projected into the external world. Some people who fail to experience mourning may escape from an outbreak of manic-depressive illness or paranoia only by a severe restriction of their emotional life which impoverishes their whole personality.

Whether some measure of mental balance can be maintained in people of this type often depends on the ways in which these various methods interact, and on their capacity to keep alive in other directions some of the love which they deny to their lost objects. Relations to people who do not in their minds come too close to the lost object, and interest in things and activities, may absorb some of this love which belonged to the lost object. Though these relations and sublimations will have some manic and paranoid qualities, they may nevertheless offer some reassurance and relief from guilt, for through them the lost loved object which has been rejected and thus again destroyed is to some extent restored and retained in the unconscious mind.

If, in our patients, analysis diminishes the anxieties of destructive and persecuting internal parents, it follows that hate and thus in turn anxieties decrease, and the patients are enabled to revise their relation to their parents—whether they be dead or alive—and to rehabilitate them to some extent even if they have grounds for actual grievances. This greater tolerance makes it possible for them to set up "good" parent-figures more securely in their minds, alongside the "bad" internal objects, or rather to mitigate the fear of these "bad" objects by the trust in "good" objects. This means enabling them to experience emotions—sorrow, guilt and grief, as well as love and trust—to go through mourning, but to overcome it, and ultimately to overcome the infantile depressive position, which they have failed to do in childhood.

To conclude. In normal mourning, as well as in abnormal mourning and in manic-depressive states, the infantile depressive position is reactivated. The complex feelings, fantasies and anxieties included under this term are of a nature which justifies my contention that the child in his early development goes through a transitory manic-depressive state as well as a state of mourning, which become modified by the infantile neurosis. With the passing of the infantile neurosis, the infantile depressive position is overcome.

The fundamental difference between normal mourning on the

one hand, and abnormal mourning and manic-depressive states on the other, is this: the manic-depressive and the person who fails in the work of mourning, though their defenses may differ widely from each other, have this in common, that they have been unable in early childhood to establish their internal "good" objects and to feel secure in their inner world. They have never really overcome the infantile depressive position. In normal mourning, however, the early depressive position, which had become revived through the loss of the loved object, becomes modified again, and is overcome by methods similar to those used by the ego in childhood. The individual is reinstating his actually lost loved object; but he is also at the same time reestablishing inside himself his first loved objects—ultimately the "good" parents—whom, when the actual loss occurred, he felt in danger of losing as well. It is by reinstating inside himself the "good" parents as well as the recently lost person, and by rebuilding his inner world, which was disintegrated and in danger, that he overcomes his grief, regains security, and achieves true harmony and peace.

NOTES

1. *Collected Papers*, Vol. IV, p. 163.
2. *Ibid.*, p. 154.
3. *Ibid.*, p. 166.
4. See p. 282. The present paper is a continuation of that paper, and much of what I have now to say will of necessity assume the conclusions I arrived at there.
5. Here I can only refer in passing to the great impetus which these anxieties afford to the development of interests and sublimations of all kinds. If these anxieties are overstrong, they may interfere with or even check intellectual development. (Cf. "A Contribution to the Theory of Intellectual Inhibition," p. 254.)
6. *The Psycho-Analysis of Children*, 1932; in particular, Chapter VIII.
7. In the same book (p. 149), referring to my view that every child passes through a neurosis differing only in degree from one individual to another, I added: "This view, which I have maintained for a number of years now, has lately received valuable support. In his book *Die Frage der Laienanalyse* (1926), Freud writes: 'Since we have learnt to see more clearly we are almost inclined to say that the occurrence of a neurosis in childhood is not the exception but the rule. It seems as though it is a thing that cannot be avoided

in the course of development from the infantile disposition to the social life of the adult'" (p. 61 — my translation).

8. At every juncture the child's feelings, fears and defenses are linked up with his libidinal wishes and fixations, and the outcome of his sexual development in childhood is always interdependent with the processes I am describing in this paper. I think that new light will be thrown on the child's libidinal development if we consider it in connection with the depressive position and the defenses used against that position. It is, however, a subject of such importance that it needs to be dealt with fully, and is therefore beyond the scope of this paper.

9. "A Contribution to the Psychogenesis of Manic-Depressive States," p. 282.

10. I have pointed out in various connections (first of all in "The Early Stages of the Oedipus Complex," p. 202) that the fear of fantastically "bad" persecutors and the belief in fantastically "good" objects are bound up with each other. Idealization is an essential process in the young child's mind, since he cannot yet cope in any other way with his fears of persecution (a result of his own hatred). Not until early anxieties have been sufficiently relieved owing to experiences which increase love and trust, is it possible to establish the all-important process of bringing together more closely the various aspects of objects (external, internal, "good" and "bad," loved and hated), and thus for hatred to become actually mitigated by love — which means a decrease of ambivalence. While the separation of these contrasting *aspects* — felt in the unconscious as contrasting *objects* — operates strongly, feelings of hatred and love are also so much divorced from each other that love cannot mitigate hatred.

The flight to the internalized "good" object, which Melitta Schmideberg (in "Psychotic Mechanisms in Cultural Development," *I.F.P.-A.*, Vol. XI, 1930) has found to be a fundamental mechanism in schizophrenia, thus also enters into the process of idealization which the young child normally resorts to in his depressive anxieties. Melitta Schmideberg has also repeatedly drawn attention to the connections between idealization and distrust of the object.

11. "A Contribution to the Psychogenesis of Manic-Depressive States," p. 282.

12. *The Psycho-Analysis of Children*, pp. 170 and 278.

13. *Ibid.*, Chapter IX.

14. These facts I think go some way toward answering Freud's question which I have quoted at the beginning of this paper: "Why this process of carrying out the behest of reality bit by bit, which is in the nature of a compromise, should be so extraordinarily painful is not at all easy to explain in terms of mental economics. It is worth noting that this pain seems natural to us."

15. "Mourning and Melancholia," *Collected Papers*, Vol. IV, p. 166.

16. Abraham writes of a situation of this kind: "We have only to reverse [Freud's] statement that 'the shadow of the lost love-object falls upon the ego' and say that in this case it was not the shadow but the bright radiance of his loved mother which was shed upon her son." (*Selected Papers*, p. 442.)

17. *Collected Papers*, Vol. IV, p. 166.

18. I have often found that processes which the patient unconsciously feels are

going on inside him are represented as something happening on top of or closely round him. By means of the well-known principle of representation by the contrary, an external happening can stand for an internal one. Whether the emphasis lies on the internal or the external situation becomes clear from the whole context — from the details of associations and the nature and intensity of affects. For instance, certain manifestations of very acute anxiety and the specific defense mechanisms against this anxiety (particularly an increase in denial of psychic reality) indicate that an internal situation predominates at the time.

19. An attack on the outside of the body often stands for one which is felt to happen internally. I have already pointed out that something represented as being on top of or tightly round the body often has the deeper meaning of being inside.

VI. DENIAL AND MOURNING

CHANNING T. LIPSON

In "Mourning and Melancholia," Freud (1917B) suggested that we could gain insight into the nature of melancholia by studying the "normal affect of mourning." As had happened before in psychoanalysis, the study of pathological phenomena shed new light in turn on our understanding of a facet of normal psychology. In this paper I shall attempt to employ this same methodology which has been so fruitful as well as valid in the past.

Mourning is the reaction to the loss of a loved one. It is a painful process which manifests itself in feelings of grief, loss of interest in the outside world, and loss of the capacity to love. The loss of object precipitates a struggle within the psyche between the reality recognition of permanent loss on the one hand, and the disinclination to abandon a libido position on the other. Withdrawal of libido takes place bit by bit, requiring a good deal of time and energy (Freud, 1917B).

Freud considered melancholia also a reaction to loss, either real or imagined. He pointed out that the response to loss in this condition was one of introjection with all its consequences. By linking mourning and melancholia and exploring them simultaneously he could discern that the nature of one's reaction to the loss of a loved object depends upon the prior relation to that object, that the elements of narcissistic object choice and ambivalence were especially significant in determining a more normal or more pathological outcome.

Abraham (1924), who considered melancholia an archaic form of mourning, observed that "in the normal process of mourning, too, the person reacts to a real object loss by effecting a temporary introjection of the loved person." In discussing the relation of identification to object loss in *The Ego and the Id,* Freud (1923) states, "It may be that this identification is the sole condition under which the id can give up its objects." These observations of Freud and Abraham have since been confirmed so frequently and so consistently that Fenichel has summarized the essence of the mourning process as consisting of two acts: "the first being the establishment of an introjection, the second the loosening of the binding to the introjected object" (1945, p. 394).

The concept that introjection is the universal response to object loss helps us to understand a wide variety of pathological grief reactions as well as many of the transient symptomatic disturbances that accompany normal mourning. We are impressed by the fact that the normal manifestations of grief, as well as such reactions as recurrent nightmares, hysterical tics, paranoid reactions, and hallucinatory psychoses, reflect the inner struggle of the ego both to escape and to master the pain of loss. Freud (1926) suggested that this pain is due to the same psychoeconomic conditions as are produced by physical pain, namely, the cumulative effect of a continuing stimulus that cannot be escaped. In the case of object loss this stimulus is the mounting cathexis of the longed-for object.

Freud (1916) also mentioned a tendency to avoid the mourning process itself. He refers (1917A) to cases in which the individual denies the loss and substitutes his own wishful fantasies for the painful reality. This attempted repudiation of the loss differs from all other forms of mourning in that it tends to bypass the whole problem of the vicissitudes of the introject. The implications of this tendency on the part of the mourning ego are best discussed in conjunction with clinical illustrations.

(1) An elderly woman was rushed to the hospital by her family following the sudden onset of a stroke. Within a few hours she died, and the attending interne immediately informed the several grown children who had remained at the hospital. Their immediate reaction was disbelief, and together they went in to see their mother. After several minutes they came from her room insisting that she was not dead, and they requested that the family physician be called. Only after the diagnosis was confirmed by a second physician did they accept the obvious reality and give vent to their intense feelings of grief.

(2) A twenty-three-year-old woman broke into violent sobbing as she told me that her mother had died two years earlier. She recalled that at the funeral she felt numb and experienced no emotion what-

soever. Her relatives admired her composure, and she herself was defiantly proud that she did not break down. She said, moreover, that her mother's death had never seemed real. Whenever she drives the hundred miles to visit her family she anticipates a pleasant day with her mother, and on each occasion she experiences intense disappointment upon discovering that her mother is not there.

The first case is a clear example of a temporary denial that is quickly abandoned in the face of reality. The second case, however, demonstrates the kind of compromise Freud described in his paper "Fetishism" (1927), namely a splitting of the ego with one part refusing to acknowledge the reality, death, and the other being fully aware of it. He states, in an apparent reference to the "Rat Man," "The patient oscillated in every situation in life between two assumptions: the one, that his father was still alive and was hindering his activities; the other, opposite one, that he was entitled to regard himself as his father's successor."*

Perhaps it is stating the obvious, but before one can establish the introject the loss has to be acknowledged. In cases of total denial this process may be postponed for years (Fleming and Altschul, 1959). Denial accompanied by simultaneous acknowledgment is the more common occurrence.

(3) A nineteen-year-old girl was interviewed five years after her mother's death. She mentioned that at the funeral she had felt that the woman in the coffin did not look like her mother. Frequently when she climbed the stairs at home she feared that she would meet her mother, and she really was not completely convinced that this had not on occasion happened. Even after five years she still entered her mother's bedroom with the expectation of finding her there.

The failure to complete mourning, accompanied by the feeling that the departed still lives, is actually quite common. In summarizing a number of articles that describe the various reactions of mourners, Bowlby (1960) reports, "All accounts dwell on the insistence with which behavior, thought, and feeling tend to remain oriented toward the lost person. Despite the knowledge that he will not return, there is a continuing sense that nonetheless he is present."

*In The Interpretation of Dreams (1900) Freud reported the following reaction of a ten-year-old boy to his father's sudden death: "I know father's dead, but what I can't understand is why he doesn't come home to supper."

It is my hypothesis that these cases of denial and ego splitting are not just a special type of reaction to loss, but have a direct relation to normal mourning, just as does melancholia. I would regard them as interruptions of mourning which permit us to observe particular stages in what is usually a fluid process, somewhat like stopping a moving picture at a particular frame.

(4) A young college girl reacted to her mother's death with depression, weight gain, and partial immobilization. Direct expressions of grief through tears and recollections were absent, and she did not connect her depression with her mother's death. After the funeral she continued to maintain her mother's bedroom as before. She would take dresses from the closet and iron them as if they were to be worn. She would discuss her current problems with her mother's photograph and feel sad that her mother didn't answer. This behavior had been going on for three months at the time she sought consultation.

After several weeks her therapist pointed out to her that she was continuing to act as if her mother still lived. Her immediate response to this was a flood of tears, followed by recollections of her mother's appearance at the time of death. A period of active mourning with affective expression, numerous reminiscences, and typical dreams followed. This was accompanied by a lifting of the depression and a resumption of her normal activities. Only then could she collect her mother's life insurance and order a headstone.

While this case clearly demonstrates the splitting of the ego, one is impressed by the fact that there has been a retardation rather than an arrest of the mourning process. The depression and weight gain suggest that some degree of introjection had taken place. Yet the girl's behavior reflected a persisting tendency to consider her mother as an external living person. The therapist's activity served to reinforce her reality testing, or at least to improve communications between the two parts of the ego.

In some cases of object loss the process of mourning is completely arrested at some intermediate stage and the entire reaction repressed. Subsequent reactivation during analysis provides a special opportunity to observe how mourning is completed by a strengthened ego.

(5) A twenty-six-year-old single woman entered analysis because of recurrent episodes of depression. During the anamnesis she men-

tioned without particular emotion that her father, a coal-miner, had been killed in a cave-in when she was nine years old. The initial phase of analysis was not unusual, as she gradually developed a clear father transference. When the first tentative transference interpretations were suggested, however, she reacted with violent denial. She asserted that the only time she was really affectionate with her father was when she was two and a half; otherwise their relationship had been distant and unimportant.

Her associations during the ensuing weeks of analysis became progressively centered on her father and the many things they did together. Something about the way she spoke of him as well as a dream involving Easter suggested to me that we were dealing with a fantasy of her father's resurrection or return that was as yet unclear. Although my ideas about this were still vague, I mentioned them to her. She became very upset, protested, and pointed out as evidence of the unlikelihood of this idea that she had never grieved for her father. Her recollection of her reaction was that she had felt she must take over for father and comfort her mother and younger sisters. She also recalled a weight gain of thirty pounds following his death.

This defensive protest, in itself revealing, did not last long, and she was able to recover many additional memories of which the following is a condensation:

She recalled being among the crowds that had assembled at the mine during the rescue operations. She was convinced that her father was safe, but, as time passed and hopes dimmed, she created a fantasied escape tunnel from which her father would emerge. After the funeral, which she attended, she continued to expect her father's return. She created new explanations of where he had gone and why his return was delayed. Many times she played out in her fantasies the dramatic scene of his sudden reappearance. Gradually these productions occupied less of her conscious fantasy life and apparently were repressed.

The elaboration of these fantasies in the analysis culminated in a sudden recollection during an analytic hour of the director of the rescue operations saying to her, "Little girl, your father is dead." Upon remembering this she was overwhelmed with grief.

Shortly after beginning analysis this woman developed periodic attacks of facial swelling that were diagnosed as angioneurotic edema. The evening following the analytic session just discussed she suffered another attack and, while reporting this to me, she recalled her father's appearance in the coffin, namely the bloated face and expanded chest. When I suggested the obvious identification with her dead father she mentioned that her facial swelling was accompanied

by a tight, painful feeling in her chest. There has been no recurrence
of the angioneurotic edema during the succeeding three years.

In retrospect it appears that the reactivation of mourning began
with the analysis; at least the repeated attacks of facial swelling
suggest this. The effect of repression was to preserve in the unconscious the fantasies of denial. With the lifting of repression these
fantasies could be reevaluated and corrected by the strengthened
adult ego, and thus permit the completion of mourning. The
analytic situation provided an opportunity to examine in detail
the relationship between denial and mourning.

As a prelude to discussing this relationship I would like to quote
the following from *An Outline of Psychoanalysis* (1940):

> We must return to our statement that the infantile ego, under the
> domination of the external world, disposes of undesirable instinctual
> demands by means of what are called repressions. We can now sup-
> plement this by a further assertion that, during the same period of
> life, the ego often enough finds itself in the position of warding off
> some claim from the external world which it feels as painful, and that
> this is effected by denying the perceptions that bring to knowledge
> such a demand on the part of reality. Denials of this kind often
> occur, and not only with fetishists; and whenever we are in a position
> to study them, they turn out to be half-measures, incomplete attempts
> at detachment from reality. The rejection is always supplemented by
> an acceptance; two contrary and independent attitudes always arise;
> and this produces the fact of a split in the ego.

Freud (1915), Moellenhoff (1939), Sterba (1948), and Wahl
(1958), among others, have pointed out that denial of the reality of
death is a general attitude in our culture. It is easily enough observed in mourners. We treat the dead in our thoughts and actions
as if they were alive. We try to make them look alive by the use of
cosmetics; we speak quietly in their presence so as not to disturb
them; we say good-bye to them, sometimes even with a kiss; we
consider their feelings in choosing an attractive and comfortable
coffin; and finally, after they are buried, we create an afterworld
in which they continue to live, and we even arrange occasional
return visits for them in ghostly form. Yet despite this active denial
we know that they are dead and we weep for them.

The loss of a loved one is potentially a traumatic situation. The ego is faced with a painful reality that it is helpless to alter. Acknowledgment of this reality threatens to flood the ego with the totality of libidinal and aggressive cathexes formerly invested in the object. Mourning is the ego's method of retarding the flood by loosening the attachment in small quantities. "What today is called grief is obviously a postponed and apportioned neutralization of a wild and self-destructive kind of affect which can still be observed in a child's panic upon the disappearance of his mother or in the uninhibited mourning reactions of primitives" (Fenichel, 1945, p. 162).

It is my conclusion, then, that the initial reaction to the loss of a loved one is denial accompanied by a splitting of the ego. This splitting of the ego is a reflection of the actual psychic state of affairs in that the ego is faced on the one hand with a highly cathected mental representation of the loved object, and on the other with an absence of perceptions of the object. The splitting is a compromise that acknowledges both realities.

We can picture what follows the splitting somewhat schematically. The instincts, still attached to the object representative, strive for gratification and repeatedly force the ego into the position of seeking the object and finding it absent. With each observation of this absence that part of the ego which has yet to acknowledge the loss experiences a degree of pain and reacts to the recognition of loss by the regressive process of introjection. Although the ultimate fate of the obect representative may be total incorporation, normally this is the result of a series of partial introjections. We know this from observing the coexistence of denial and introjection as well as the transitory partial identifications that accompany normal mourning. Concurrent with this series of partial introjections is a parallel series of partial detachments from the introject. This is suggested by the gradual diminution of sadness and the slow renewal of energy that take place during mourning.

Introjection is an attempt to preserve the object, but it is also a step toward giving it up. In fact it does not take place until the loss is acknowledged. Denial is also an attempt to preserve the object, but perhaps its more basic function is to preserve the ego.

REFERENCES

ABRAHAM, KARL (1924). "A Short Study of the Development of the Libido, Viewed in the Light of Mental Disorders." *Selected Papers* (London: Hogarth), p. 435.

BOWLBY, JOHN (1960). "Grief and Mourning in Infancy and Early Childhood," *Psychoanal. Study Child,* 15, p. 17.

FENICHEL, OTTO (1945). *The Psychoanalytic Theory of Neurosis* (New York: Norton).

FLEMING, J., and ALTSCHUL, S. (1959). "Activation of Mourning and Growth by Psychoanalysis," presented to Chicago Psychoanal. Soc. Abstract in *Bull. Philadelph. Assoc. Psychoanal.,* 9.

FREUD, S. (1900). *The Interpretation of Dreams.* S.E., 4, p. 254 n.

—— (1915). "Thoughts for the Times on War and Death," *S.E.* 14, pp. 289–300.

—— (1916). "On Transience." *S.E.* 14.

—— (1917A). "A Metapsychological Supplement to the Theory of Dreams." *S.E.* 14, pp. 233–235.

—— (1917B). "Mourning and Melancholia." *S.E.* 14.

—— (1923). *The Ego and the Id. S.E.* 19, p. 29.

—— (1926). *Inhibitions, Symptoms and Anxiety. S.E.* 20, pp. 170–172.

—— (1927). "Fetishism." *S.E.* 21.

—— (1940). *An Outline of Psychoanalysis* (New York: Norton, 1949) pp. 118–119.

MOELLENHOFF, F. (1939). "Ideas of Children about Death: A Preliminary Study." *Bull. Menninger Clinic,* 3.

STERBA, R. (1948). "On Hallowe'en." *Amer. Imago,* 5.

WAHL, C. W. (1958). "The Fear of Death." *Bull. Menninger Clinic,* 22.

VII. GRIEF REACTIONS IN LATER LIFE

KARL STERN,
GWENDOLYN M. WILLIAMS,
AND
MIGUEL PRADOS

The gerontologic unit within the Department of Psychiatry at McGill University has been running an old-age counselling service since 1945. A description of this type of service and the main problems involved has been given on previous occasions (1, 2). One of the most frequent situations with which one has to deal in this age group is that of bereavement. This is probably accentuated by the fact that the patients seen in the counselling service are members of the indigent population. In such a socially and economically selected group the patient comes to the attention of a social agency for the first time when he or she loses a marital partner or some other family member. In the following study an attempt is made to draw attention to certain features of grief reactions that are particularly striking within this age group and that may differ in character from grief reactions in younger age groups.

Subjects

The present observations were made on 25 subjects, one of whom was male and 24 of whom were female. The age at the time of interview varies from fifty-three to seventy. As has been indicated (1), the problems encountered in old age can only be artificially differentiated from those of the involutional period. Therefore, in this study the age range is greater and the lower age limit is fifty.

Method

A social history is taken by the social worker before the psychiatrist sees the patient. A systematic psychiatric history is taken in the first interview, which is followed by a varying number of informal interviews. For reasons previously given (1), even the first interview has to be kept "free" so that the patient does not have the feeling of a systematic "history taking." The facts have to be compiled gradually during several interviews, as well as from the history taken by the social worker.

Observations

A composite picture of these cases presents itself as follows. There is a dearth of overt mental manifestations of grief or of conscious guilt feelings. On the other hand, there is a preponderance of somatic illness. In some cases the time relationship between the onset or accentuation of these somatic illnesses and the time of bereavement is quite obvious. The image of the deceased undergoes peculiar changes in the consciousness of the mourner; the idealization commonly encountered during the process of grief sometimes assumes bizarre degrees. In contrast to this there frequently develops an irrational hostility toward living persons, particularly in the patient's immediate environment. Here there is also a time relationship between the onset of the hostility and the time of bereavement in some cases.

The features are best illustrated by some case examples.

> A woman of fifty-nine (Mrs. A. C.), who had lost her husband two years before she was first seen, developed arthritis at the time of his death. She had an operation for prolapse of the bladder on the day of the anniversary of his death. "Coming out" of the operation she developed a pain in her right arm that since has "spread all over."
>
> A man of fifty-nine (Mr. J. S.) developed breathlessness and a large amount of sputum within the year following his wife's death, which had occurred six years before the first interview. At that time bronchiectases were diagnosed.
>
> A woman of sixty-three (Mrs. I. T.) who had lost her husband six years before the first interview, suffered three accidents within four years, always when in domestic employment. On one occasion she slipped and broke her wrist while the family for whom she was working was preparing the house for Christmas.

A woman of sixty-eight (Mrs. E. G.) was seen five months after the death of her husband. The latter had given up work five to six years before his death because of "heart trouble." During the six months before he died he was unable to hold his urine. His wife nursed him during this time. Three months after she had begun to nurse him she developed diarrhea. When asked how she reacted to her husband's death she said that it still came as a shock to her. However, this was stated without any sign of emotional depth. Six weeks after her husband's death she had an intestinal operation for her diarrhea. A surgeon told her afterwards that "the large bowels and the small bowels were intertwined and that is what caused the pain." When first seen she still complained of this diarrhea, of precordial pain, and undue fatigability. Since the time of her husband's death she had lost 15 lbs. She had no emotional complaints except for "worrying about everything." She looked serious but laughed quite readily at times and was able to see a joke. The conversation lacked spontaneity and all information had to be gained by specific questions.

One woman of sixty-three (Mrs. I. R.) was admitted to the Allan Memorial Institute with the typical picture of a senile dementia. Interviews of the relatives revealed the fact that her organic cerebral syndrome set in immediately following her husband's death. This time relationship was stated independently by several relatives.

This woman was born in Montreal. Her father died at the age of eighty-four of cancer. He was an engineer and had emigrated from England. Her mother died of cancer at the age of eighty. The patient was the third of ten children of whom six were still living at the time of interview. Two children died in infancy of meningitis, one sister died of typhoid fever, one brother died of cancer, and another brother had been in a mental hospital for the last ten years. After completing high school she took a business course and worked for more than ten years with an insurance company.

At the age of twenty-eight she married, and her husband was approximately the same age. Her relationship with him seems to have been a very dependent one. She said that arguments were her fault because she was "such a little snip." She had very high praise for his thoughtfulness, his ability at the office, and his musical talent: "I don't like to brag but . . ." The main social activities of their life were centered about the church and the choir, for which her husband was the organist. He was employed by an insurance firm. They entertained friends in their home. She could not have children and said that she now felt inadequate. She treated her nephew "as my son."

According to information obtained from her sister, the patient had never been considered a strong person. Twice she had travelled to England because she felt "terribly worn down" after the death of a near relative. These trips made her feel much better. She had had a gynecological operation many years ago. She had a gastroenterostomy for the relief of an obstructive ulcer. She had had pleurisy and bronchitis the two winters previous to the death of her husband.

In August 1949 her husband died suddenly as the result of an accident; while doing some house painting he fell on a picket fence and his lung was pierced. Following his death she became restless and anxious; at the same time it was noticed that she became forgetful, increasingly disoriented, and negligent in her everyday work. In October 1950 she was admitted to the Allan Memorial Institute.

She was a short, thin and pale woman, with a mild facial asymmetry. She would move restlessly about the ward, repeating over and over that she was a nuisance to everybody, that she could not understand why people were so kind to her, and that she ought to have her glasses fixed. Physical examination revealed diminished hearing in the left ear, diminished vision in the left eye, a sluggish right pupillary response, an equivocal plantar reflex on the right, bradycardia (50), and retinal arteriosclerosis.

Interview: (What is your name?) "Ivy, a plant. . . . I was the first girl, so they thought they had to give me a flower name. . . . You have a pretty view up here. . . . My husband and I used to go for lovely walks in the fall. . . . Do you have a son? . . . A doctor who examined my eyes had a son here, that's why I thought you might have a son...."

(What is wrong with you?) "Just if I could see, read . . . it's my eyes."

(How long have you had this?) "It dates back to childhood. I think I had a fall when I was a child, I think it's that what causes all the trouble. . . ."

(Is there anything else wrong with you? You would not be taken into this place on account of your eyesight.) "I don't know. . . . They told me to come here, that's all."

(How do you sleep?) "I sleep fairly well since I got over the shock. It was a month, I don't know exactly."

(How is your appetite?) "Thank you, that's improved."

(How is your memory?) "The first little while after the shock I didn't remember so well."

(What would you say is the date today?) "I don't care. . . . I didn't follow it up. (Looks through the window.) Oh, I *do* know, it's November sixth, my birthday." (Correct)

(What year is it?) "Oh, I don't have any occasion, I didn't write letters. . . . Oh, I give up, I'm half asleep anyway."

(Would you say it is closer to 1948 or to 1938?) "I would rather say it's 1940 something than 1930 something."

(Examiner had introduced himself twice before. "What is my name?") "I don't think I heard it." (Examiner repeats his name.) "Oh yes, you told me so. I thought I had only my eyes to be tested."

(What was the shock you mentioned?) "I made a great mistake. My brother-in-law said all the time to keep it up. . . . That's why my side is sore all the time, I feel tight here. I don't get any breath. It's dreadful to be alone in the house. You know we were very near, we had no children. That silence in the house, how can I stand it? My brother didn't understand me (cries). You see, my husband was musical, we often had the choir in the house. When the accident took place he had three different offers to play the organ."

She gave contradictory reports as to the actual time of the accident. Her retention was severely impaired on counting tests(3). She showed considerable stability in her defects during several examinations within two weeks.*

The following examples illustrate the actual attitude toward the lost person; all "dark" features are blotted out and the deceased becomes transfigured in an unreal way.

A woman of sixty (Mrs. E. D.) who had lost her husband three years before the first interview complained of "feeling bad" in a busy or noisy environment. Her sleep was poor, appetite varied, digestion was irregular. "Sometimes I don't feel too bad, at other times I feel like dying." She described her husband as a "wonderful man." Actually he had been an alcoholic who deserted her on several occasions and was cruel when intoxicated. There were notes in the record at the Family Welfare Association to the effect that she had come running for protection and help. In successive interviews she gave a glowing picture of her husband, and when finally confronted with the facts she denied them.

A similar situation existed in the case of a woman of sixty-one (Mrs. H. W.), who was seen in private practice. She had lost her husband seven years before the first interview. This woman referred to her deceased husband in terms that struck the examiner as almost fantastic glorification. Moreover, she invoked his name in connection with any, even trivial, decision she had to make. Remarks such as, "Walter would want me to do this . . ." or ". . . would not want me to

*The authors wish to thank Dr. D. Ewen Cameron for allowing them to use his test results in this case.

do that," occurred frequently. She had a villa in one of the most beautiful spots of Sweden and spent part of every year there. Several rooms of the villa remained untouched, as if she were dealing with a shrine in his memory. The history taken from her son and her daughter revealed that the husband had been a psychopath with sadistic features. He had retired early in life, around the age of forty, living on his ample income. Every morning he would sit at his writing desk and compose an exact timetable of duties for each member of the family. This included physical exercises, open air walks, etc., even for the Parkinsonian mother-in-law, who frequently pleaded not to have to go for walks on cold days but was forced to do so just the same. He carried on an affair with the children's governess for many years, and would bring well-known dancers and actresses as "guests" into the home. Our informants told us that the patient had not only known about these things, but it seems that her husband made sure that she would know about them.

Another trend observed in our group was toward self-isolation, and of hostility against people in the bereaved person's surroundings. In fact, at times the immediate reason for which the social worker brought the client to the attention of the old age counselling service was precisely because he or she had "turned against" other roomers in the house, or against a member of the family, usually of the same sex as the deceased.

A woman of sixty-one (Mrs. M. B.), who was first seen two years after her husband's death, complained of insomnia and anorexia. "I've had a sour stomach all my life. Milk, if it is not cooked properly, doesn't agree with me." She said that she had cried a good deal since her husband's death. "If it were not for crying I'd be dead. It's the only thing that relieves me."

At the age of twenty-seven she had married a man ten years her senior. She said that she had known her husband since childhood because he came into her house." For several years before his death he suffered from "amnesia" (described what appeared to be senile dementia) and she apparently had a difficult time with him. "He wanted to go out all the time. One night he went out in his underwear and with his straw hat on." The last six months of his life he was in a mental institution. They had one child, a married daughter. After his death, our patient had a terrible quarrel with her son-in-law. When asked why, she was rather vague: "I did not like the way he acted. . . . He is rather a nervous man himself."

The private patient mentioned above developed a marked hostility against her son-in-law shortly after her husband's death. She described him as a cruel man who held her daughter in subjugation. Actually the daughter was happily married and, according to the latter as well as her son, the picture she gave of her son-in-law was completely distorted and would actually have fitted her husband.

Treatment

None of the cases described here was psychotic, nor was the depression of such a degree that electric shock treatment or hospitalization was necessary. The mechanisms of transference are largely modified in this age group (2). In view of the numerous somatic illnesses it must be emphasized that the patient needs to feel that the psychiatrist keeps close track and shows genuine interest in all medical and surgical procedures.

All channels toward sublimation have to be carefully exploited. The private patient (Mrs. H. W.) whose husband had been "idealized" in such an incongruous fashion developed a strong hero-worship of her minister, and began much church activity and community work, and is now on good terms with her son-in-law.

A large part of the therapy in the cases described consists of manipulating the environment. The mechanisms of hostility and self-isolation have to be interpreted to the relatives. Whenever possible the patient himself should be led up to the point of insight. In the cases of irrational hostility directed toward a member of the family the hostility disappeared during the course of the interviews.

Discussion

Reactions of grief and mourning are so important from a clinical point of view that they have been studied intensively(4–9). Most of these investigations are based on psychoanalytic concepts. The one persistent trend apparent in all these papers is the one implied in Freud's original study (4), and best formulated in the observation by Helene Deutsch (5), namely, that the "work" of mourning must be viewed in the light of the psychoanalytic theory of libido. This theory is based on an analogy between the "conservation" of libido on one hand, and the law of conservation of energy on the other.

From a review of the literature it appears that grief reactions in later life have never been studied systematically. If we look at the most important features observed in our group, namely, the relative paucity of conscious guilt feelings, the tendency toward a replacement of the emotional grief reaction by somatic equivalents, the distortion of the image of the deceased in the direction of some unreal glorification, the tendency to self-isolation and hostility toward surviving members of the family or toward friends, it seems that they all lend themselves to an interpretation along the lines evolved in the psychoanalytic literature. Helene Deutsch (5) explained the absence of mourning in children on the basis of the assumption that the child's ego is too weak to carry out the "work" of mourning. Grief would endanger the ego at that stage to such a degree that the child has an immediate scotoma for the loss. However, she contends that the process of grief must be completed later. Now it has been stated that old age is characterized by a weakening of the strength of the ego; on this basis it has been assumed that involutional depressions are due to the fact that dynamic forces emanating from the superego are relatively prevalent during the involution (10). This relative strengthening of the superego is made possible by the waning of the ego in the aging person.

If this theory is correct one should, at first sight, assume that conscious guilt, or a tendency toward delusions of guilt, should be found more frequently in old than in young bereaved persons. Our observations, however, seem to indicate the opposite. In order to explain this apparent discrepancy, namely, between a greater tendency to overt guilt in later life melancholias and the comparative absence of guilt in states of mourning, we have to consider the following. Under certain circumstances the older person is more ready to "channel" material that would produce overt emotional conflict into somatic illness. It is interesting to note in this connection Cobb's observation that the correlation between psychogenic trauma and rheumatoid arthritis became greater as the age of the investigated patients increased (11). Something analogous was observed in the first hundred clients of our old age counselling service (1). It would be the subject of a special study to decide whether these somatic illnesses represent a tendency toward self-punishment or an expression of the death wish and an identification with the deceased. However, it is safe to assume that the aging organism is biologically more ready for somatic equivalents of depressions. Even the senile dementia observed in one of our cases obviously represented such a flight into the somatic. It is generally known that degenerative cerebral disease can be enhanced or precipitated by emotional factors. Kral (12) showed that in elderly inmates of concentration camps there were not more affective psychotic disorders than would be expected in a control group but there was, under emotional stress, a definite tendency toward precipitation of organic senile psychoses. Incidentally, it is interesting to study the verbal productions of our senile patient from the point of view of the symbolic connotations of the psychogenic factor. She believes that she is in the hospital to have her eyesight tested. This may be interpreted, as in the case of a hysterical blindness, as representing her wish "not to see." Moreover, she thinks that her illness is due to a fall she had during childhood. On another occasion she points at the side of her chest and indicates that it hurts in there. There is little doubt that the "fall" and the pain in her side are associated with the mode of death of her husband who had been killed by falling on a picket fence and piercing his lung.

The most extensive and systematic study of grief reactions (Lindemann (8)) was carried out chiefly on the bereaved persons after a disaster with violent death. This kind of death has unconscious symbolic connotations that, for obvious reasons, lend themselves more to the formation of ideas of guilt. In elderly people the death of the deceased has often been expected over a long time; there is frequently a history of nursing the sick person for a long period before death; the bereaved person is at an age at which he is preparing for death—in other words, contrary to situations like those described by Lindemann, there is more opportunity to identify with the deceased rather than feel guilty toward him.

This may also explain the tendency toward distortion. Helene Deutsch (5) emphasized that ambivalence toward the deceased is the most difficult conflict to master during the reaction of mourning. In our cases we saw a tendency to preserve an image of the deceased consisting only of light without shadow. We might say that the shadow is buried, or in those cases in which the shadow is not repressed it is projected onto a living person. This would explain the irrational hostility toward a living member of the family.

In fact, the description that the bereaved gives of the relative toward whom he displays hostility may correspond surprisingly to the objectionable features of the deceased. In any case, the ambivalence is handled by splitting the image of the deceased into two. This mechanism is suggestive of an ego defense. To work through the ambivalence on a conscious level would be too great a strain. In purifying the image of the deceased to an unreal degree, the bereaved fulfils narcissistic needs that are urgent at this stage of life and avoids the intolerable stress of overt hostility.

Thus, we can tentatively explain all the phenomena observed here on the basis of defense against dynamic forces that would be destructive to a weakened ego. Apart from this, it is possible that the "somatic equivalents" of grief reactions are facilitated by identification with the deceased and the death wish of the mourner.

Summary

Grief reactions in later life have been studied in 25 subjects, 23 of whom attended an old-age counselling service. The most striking features in this group were: a relative paucity of overt grief and of conscious guilt feelings, a preponderance of somatic illness precipitated or accentuated by the bereavement; a tendency to extreme exaggeration of the common idealization of the deceased with a blotting-out of all "dark" features; a tendency to self-isolation and to hostility against some living person. These features are discussed in the light of the psychoanalytic theories of mourning and depressions in general, as applied to the psychological dynamics of later life. A brief outline of the management of these cases is given.

BIBLIOGRAPHY

1. STERN, KARL. "Observations in an Old Age Counselling Center." *J. Gerontol,* 3 (1948): 48.
2. STERN, KARL. "Problems Encountered in an Old Age Counselling Center." In *Problems of Aging.* New York: Josiah Macy, Jr. Foundation, (1950).
3. CAMERON, D. EWEN, and FELDMAN, F. "The Measurement of Remembering." *Am. J. Psychiat.,* 100 (May 1944): 7.

4. FREUD, SIGMUND. "Mourning and Melancholia." *Collected Papers* IV. 10: 152.
5. DEUTSCH, HELENE. "Absence of Grief." *Psychoanal. Quart.*, 6 (1937): 12.
6. KLEIN, MELANIE. "Mourning and Manic-Depressive States." *Internat. J. Psychoanal.*, 21 (1940): 125.
7. COBB, STANLEY, and LINDEMANN, ERICH. "Neuropsychiatric Observations after the Cocoanut Grove Fire." *Ann. Surg.*, 117 (June 1943): 814.
8. LINDEMANN, ERICH. "Symptomatology and Management of Acute Grief." *Am. J. Psychiat.*, 101 (Sept. 1944): 141.
9. ROSENBAUM, MILTON. "Emotional Aspects of Wartime Separations." *Family*, 24 (1944): 337.
10. PEARSON, GERALD H. J. "An Interpretative Study of Involutional Depression." *Am. J. Psychiat.*, 85 (Sept. 1928): 289.
11. COBB, S., et al. "Environmental Factors in Rheumatoid Arthritis." *J.A.M.A.*, 113 (1939): 668.
12. KRAL, V. A. "Psychiatric Observations of Chronic Stress." *Am. J. Psychiat.*, 108 (Sept. 1951): 185.